Lecture Notes in Computer Science 14668

Founding Editors

Gerhard Goos
Juris Hartmanis

The series Lecture Notes in Computer Science (LNCS), including its subseries Lecture Notes in Artificial Intelligence (LNAI) and Lecture Notes in Bioinformatics (LNBI), has established itself as a medium for the publication of new developments in computer science and information technology research, teaching, and education.

LNCS enjoys close cooperation with the computer science R & D community, the series counts many renowned academics among its volume editors and paper authors, and collaborates with prestigious societies. Its mission is to serve this international community by providing an invaluable service, mainly focused on the publication of conference and workshop proceedings and postproceedings. LNCS commenced publication in 1973.

Ujjwal Baid · Reuben Dorent · Sylwia Malec ·
Monika Pytlarz · Ruisheng Su ·
Navodini Wijethilake · Spyridon Bakas ·
Alessandro Crimi
Editors

Brainlesion: Glioma, Multiple Sclerosis, Stroke and Traumatic Brain Injuries

9th International Workshop, BrainLes 2023
and 3rd International Workshop, SWITCH 2023
Held in Conjunction with MICCAI 2023
Vancouver, BC, Canada, October 8 and 12, 2023
Revised Selected Papers

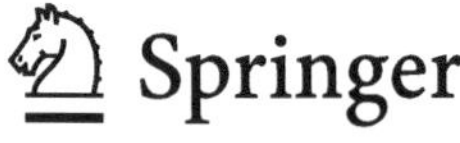

Editors
Ujjwal Baid
Indiana University School of Medicine
Indianapolis, IN, USA

Sylwia Malec
Indiana University School of Medicine
Indianapolis, IN, USA

Ruisheng Su
Eindhoven University of Technology
Eindhoven, The Netherlands

Spyridon Bakas
Indiana University School of Medicine
Indianapolis, IN, USA

Reuben Dorent
Harvard Medical School
Boston, MA, USA

Monika Pytlarz
Sano – Centre for Computational Personalised Medicine International Research Foundation
Kraków, Poland

Navodini Wijethilake
King's College London
London, UK

Alessandro Crimi
Sano – Centre for Computational Personalised Medicine International Research Foundation
Kraków, Poland

ISSN 0302-9743 ISSN 1611-3349 (electronic)
Lecture Notes in Computer Science
ISBN 978-3-031-76159-1 ISBN 978-3-031-76160-7 (eBook)
https://doi.org/10.1007/978-3-031-76160-7

This Springer imprint is published by the registered company Springer Nature Switzerland AG
The registered company address is: Gewerbestrasse 11, 6330 Cham, Switzerland

Preface

This volume contains articles from the Brain Lesion workshop (BrainLes 2023), as well as the Stroke Workshop on Imaging and Treatment CHallenges (SWITCH 2023). These events were held in conjunction with the Medical Image Computing and Computer Assisted Intervention (MICCAI) conference on the 8th–12th of October 2023 in Vancouver, Canada.

The presented manuscripts describe the research of computational scientists and clinical researchers working on brain lesions, and specifically glioma, multiple sclerosis, cerebral stroke, traumatic brain injuries, vestibular schwannoma, and white matter hyperintensities of presumed vascular origin. This compilation does not claim to provide a comprehensive understanding from all points of view; however, the authors present their latest advances in segmentation, disease prognosis, stroke diagnosis and treatment, and other applications to the clinical context.

The volume is divided into two chapters: The first chapter comprises the accepted paper submissions to the BrainLes workshop, and the second chapter contain a selection of papers regarding methods presented at SWITCH.

The aim of the **first chapter**, focusing on the accepted **BrainLes workshop submissions**, is to provide an overview of new advances in medical image analysis in all the aforementioned brain pathologies. It brings together researchers from the medical image analysis domain, neurologists, and radiologists working on at least one of these diseases. The aim is to consider neuroimaging biomarkers used for one disease applied to the other diseases. This session did not have a specific dataset to be used.

The **second chapter** contains a selection of papers from the **SWITCH 2023** challenge participants. The SWITCH workshop focused on imaging related to stroke diagnosis and treatment. The main goals of the workshop were 1) to introduce the clinical background of challenges/opportunities related to imaging for stroke that are relevant for researchers working in the MICCAI field, and 2) to stimulate discussion and ideas exchange. In the workshop, keynotes were delivered by clinical experts in stroke imaging and treatment, and accepted works were presented by authors. The challenges in stroke imaging were addressed by three clinical keynote speakers, Menon Bijoy (University of Calgary) on computer-aided diagnosis in acute ischemic stroke, Pascal Mosimann (University of Toronto) on remote neurovascular interventions, and Jonas Richiardi (University of Lausanne) on MRI in stroke. The accepted papers focus on AI-based detection and segmentation of stroke lesions and function outcome prediction in acute ischemic stroke. The organizers of the SWITCH workshop would like to express their sincere thanks to the keynote speakers, the authors of the contributed papers, and the attendees of the workshops.

We heartily hope that this volume will promote further exciting computational research on brain-related pathologies.

The organizers,

Ujjwal Baid
Spyridon Bakas
Alessandro Crimi
Reuben Dorent
Sylwia Malec
Monika Pytlarz
Ruisheng Su
Navodini Wijethilake

Organization

BrainLes Organizing Committee

Ujjwal Baid	Indiana University, USA
Spyridon Bakas	Indiana University, USA
Alessandro Crimi	Sano Centre for Computational Medicine, Poland
Sylwia Malec	Sano Centre for Computational Medicine, Poland
Monika Pytlarz	Sano Centre for Computational Medicine, Poland

BrainLes Program Committee

Sanyukta Adap	Indiana University, USA
Bhakti Baheti	Indiana University, USA
Ujjwal Baid	Indiana University, USA
Sindhuja Tirumalai Govindarajan	University of Pennsylvania, USA
Cemal Koba	Sano Centre for Computational Medicine, Poland
Florian Kofler	Technical University of Munich, Germany
Hugo Kuijf	University Medical School of Utrecht, The Netherlands
Andreas Mang	University of Houston, USA
Siddhesh Thakur	Indiana University, USA
Diana Waldmannstetter	Technical University of Munich, Germany
Benedikt Wiestler	Technical University of Munich, Germany

Stroke Workshop on Imaging and Treatment Challenges (SWITCH)

Jeroen Bertels	KU Leuven, Belgium
Adrian Dalca	MIT and MGH, Harvard Medical School, USA
Danny Ruijters	TU Eindhoven, The Netherlands
Ruisheng Su	Erasmus MC, The Netherlands
Theo van Walsum	Erasmus MC, The Netherlands
Roland Wiest	Support Center for Advanced Neuroimaging, Inselspital Bern, Switzerland
Anke Wouters	KU Leuven, Belgium

Contents

BrainLes

SWITCH

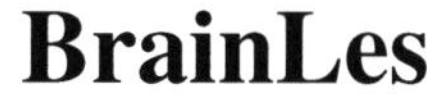
BrainLes

Detection of Onset Time for Acute Ischemic Stroke Based on Multi-scale Features and Cross-Attention

Bao Yang[1], Peng Yang[1], Zifeng Qiu[1], Yueyan Bian[2], JiaQiang Li[1], Xiang Dong[1], Junlong Qu[1], Qi Yang[2,3](✉), and Baiying Lei[1](✉)

[1] Guangdong Key Laboratory for Biomedical Measurements and Ultrasound Imaging, National-Regional Key Technology Engineering Laboratory for Medical Ultrasound, School of Biomedical Engineering, Shenzhen University Medical school, Shenzhen 518060, China
leiby@szu.edu.cn

[2] Department of Radiology, Beijing Chaoyang Hospital, Capital Medical University, Beijing, China
yangyangqiqi@gmail.com

[3] Laboratory for Clinical Medicine, Capital Medical University, Beijing, China

Abstract. Acute ischemic stroke (AIS) is a cerebral disease that can lead to severe brain tissue damage and even death. The optimal treatment window for AIS is within 6 h since time since stroke (TSS). Computed tomography perfusion (CTP) provides crucial brain-related information and plays a significant role in the diagnosis and treatment of AIS. However, CTP data poses challenges due to its small sample size, high dimensionality, and the heterogeneity and interdependence among the four types of perfusion images. To effectively utilize CTP data for accurately assessing the time window and preventing disease progression, we propose a classification model based on multi-scale feature fusion and cross-attention mechanisms tailored to the clinical characteristics of CTP. Specifically, we employ a multi-scale feature extraction (MFE) blocks to combine features from various scales and utilize a cross-attention fusion (CAF) module to merge complementary features. Finally, the multi-head pooling attention (MPA) is employed to further learn feature information and obtain as much critical information as possible. To validate the effectiveness of our proposed approach on a hospital's private dataset, we conduct a 5-fold cross-validation strategy. Experimental results demonstrate that our method exhibits superiority in the TSS classification task and possesses high robustness.

Keywords: Acute ischemic stroke · Time since stroke onset · Multi-scale feature extraction · Cross-attention

1 Introduction

Acute ischemic stroke (AIS) is a condition caused by insufficient blood supply to part of the brain [1], leading to a cascade of reactions. If the brain tissue is deprived of oxygen for more than 60 to 90 s, it stops functioning, and irreversible damage may occur within a few

U. Baid et al. (Eds.): BrainLes 2023/SWITCH 2023, LNCS 14668, pp. 3–12, 2024.
https://doi.org/10.1007/978-3-031-76160-7_1

hours, possibly leading to brain tissue death [2]. According to the 2019 International Stroke Treatment Guidelines, ischemic stroke patients without contraindications can receive intravenous thrombolytic therapy within 4.5 h from symptom onset. Patients with large vessel occlusion can undergo thrombectomy to open the blocked blood vessels, with the optimal time for thrombectomy being within 6 h from symptom onset [3, 4]. A treatment window with a time since stroke snset (TSS) of less than 6 h is considered a safe and appropriate timeframe for intervention. Therefore, accurately determining the onset time of stroke in patients is crucial for initiating the next steps of treatment. The diagnosis of AIS can be facilitated through computed tomography perfusion (CTP) imaging, which provides personalized selection criteria.

To classify the affected brain regions, CTP scans utilize dedicated software to generate four perfusion maps: cerebral blood flow (CBF), cerebral blood volume (CBV), mean transit time (MTT), and peak response time (Tmax) [5]. These maps represent the regions of the stroke core, penumbra, and mirrored penumbra. CTP is more easily accessible for patients and much faster than other imaging techniques such as Magnetic Resonance Imaging (MRI) [6]. At the same time, it can provide doctors with more comprehensive cerebral blood flow information, allowing them to assess relevant information about ischemic penumbra areas and infarct core regions, providing various data for clinical purposes [7]. Therefore, we utilize the relevant information obtained from CTP images of the brain to determine whether the TSS is less than 6 h for the patients.

With the advancement of Artificial Intelligence, machine learning and deep learning have been widely employed for the analysis of neuroimaging data. In recent years, researchers have also attempted to apply machine learning and deep learning methods to TSS classification. For instance, Govindarajan et al. [8] proposed a stroke classification prototype that combines text mining tools and machine learning algorithms. Machine learning algorithms, trained appropriately, are utilized for classification. Garg *et al.* [9] integrated natural language processing of electronic health records with machine learning methods to achieve automated classification. Mittermeier *et al.* [10]developed a novel convolutional neural network to extract spatial and temporal features from time-resolved imaging data for stroke classification. Dourado *et al.* [11] proposed an automated method for detecting ischemic stroke using computer-aided decision systems for MRI diffusion-weighted image sequences, *Neethi et al.* [12] introduced a 3D fully convolutional classification model for identifying stroke cases from non-contrast computed tomography images.

The aforementioned classification methods based on machine learning and deep learning typically suffer from the following drawbacks. Firstly, they heavily rely on textual information while overlooking the importance of medical imaging. Secondly, the limited sample size and high dimensionality of CTP data can lead to overfitting issues, resulting in the inability to learn critical features and convergence problems. Some existing TSS classification methods using CTP data employ very deep network models, which are prone to overfitting and lack generalization capabilities, while not fully exploiting the supplementary information present in the data [13, 14].

Therefore, in this study, we propose a classification model for AIS patients' TSS based on multi-scale feature fusion and cross-attention mechanism. Specifically, we first use a multi-scale feature extraction (MFE) blocks to extract multi-scale information features from the images. Then, a cross-attention fusion (CAF) module [15] is employed to integrate complementary features. Finally, we employ the multi-head pooling attention (MPA) method to further learn feature information, extracting as much important information as possible and selecting the most discriminative features for classifying whether the onset time window of the patients exceeds 6 h.

Our main contributions are as follows:

- The paper proposes a framework that utilizes MFE blocks and CAF to effectively capture multi-scale and complementary information from CTP data, thereby improving the accuracy of stroke diagnosis.
- The MFE blocks is employed to extract multi-scale information features from CTP images, which enhances the diagnostic performance of the model.
- The CAF is introduced to extract complementary information from different perfusion images.
- We applied our method to a private dataset and conducted extensive experiments to validate its reliability. The results demonstrated that our approach exhibits a certain level of robustness and effectiveness.

2 Methodology

2.1 Method Overview

The main framework of the method is illustrated in Fig. 1. The TSS classification approach in this chapter is a network model based on multi-scale feature extraction and cross-attention fusion. Specifically, each perfusion map's feature extraction is independently carried out by four identical encoders. The MFE blocks is used to capture different-scale details and fuse them, enhancing the acquisition of correlated information sets at different scales. In the final stages, the CAF module is utilized to globally integrate spatial correlations of the perfusion map features, strengthening the complementary feature interaction fusion between each perfusion map. Finally, before feeding the learned feature information into the fully connected layer of the network, the features are encoded and then further learned using the MPA, which consolidates the latent tensor sequences. Ultimately, the selected features are fed into the fully connected layer to achieve TSS classification.

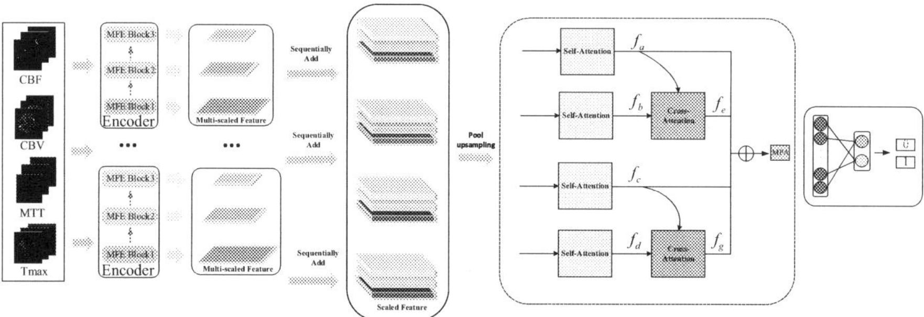

Fig. 1. Illustration of the proposed method.

2.2 Multi-scale Feature Extraction Block

Considering that the perfusion maps contain information features at different scales, we employ a multi-scale feature extraction module to fuse the perfusion map features. The structure of this module is illustrated in Fig. 2.

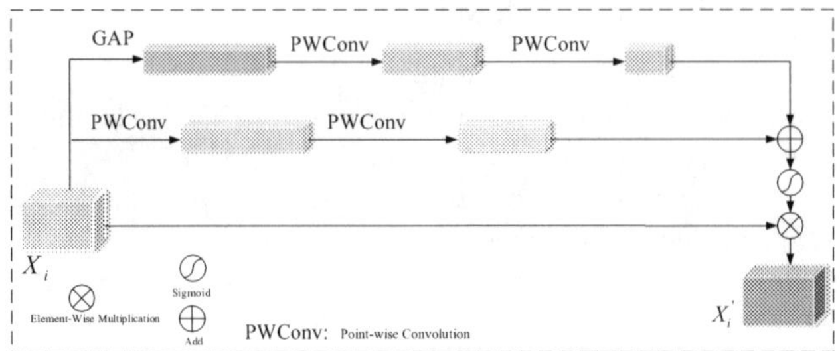

Fig. 2. Illustration of MFE. Setting different spatial pooling sizes allows for focusing on interaction feature information from multiple scales in the channel dimension.

By setting different spatial pooling sizes, it is possible to focus on the interactive feature information at multiple scales in the channel dimension, aggregating both local and global features. To keep it as lightweight as possible, the local context is incorporated into the global context of the attention module. This is achieved by utilizing point-wise convolution to interact with each spatial position through point-wise channel interaction, enabling the integration of local information. Let $X_i (i = 1,2,3,4)$ denote the input features for each branch, where i represents the i-th modality. The computation of the local channel features is defined as follows:

$$L(X_i) = PWConv(ReLu(PWConv(GAP(X_i)))) \tag{1}$$

The kernel sizes of $PWConv$ are $\frac{C}{r} \times C \times 1 \times 1 \times 1$ and $C \times \frac{C}{r} \times 1 \times 1 \times 1$, respectively. The computation of global channel features is demoted as follows:

$$G(X_i) = PWConv(ReLu(PWConv(X_i))) \tag{2}$$

The final feature X_i' is computed as follows:

$$X_i' = X_i \oplus \sigma(L(X_i) \oplus G(X_i)) \tag{3}$$

For each scale of information features, we adopt a progressive addition approach, similar to the operation in Feature Pyramid Network. We upsample the scale information and then perform element-wise addition to combine the features.

2.3 Cross-Attention Fusion Module

The fusion of complementary information between infusion maps considers the correlation of global information among different infusion maps. To achieve this, we use the self-attention mechanism [16] and cross-attention [15] from the transformer architecture to extract global information and fuse complementary information, as illustrated in Fig. 1. Specifically, the output features at each stage are denoted as $X_{ij}(i = 4{,}5; j = 1{,}2, 3{,}4)$, where i represents the feature output from the i-th stage and j represents the j-th modality. Similar to the previous works applying transformers to images [17–20], we treat the intermediate feature maps of each modality as sets rather than patches and consider each element in the set as a token. At this point, each token incorporates information from all tokens of the four branches. To achieve data fusion between infusion maps [21], we use f_a, f_b, f_c and f_d as inputs to the cross-attention computation block. We treat f_a and f_c as auxiliary information and embed them into the features of f_b and f_d through cross-attention. Specifically, we replace the keys and values with f_a and f_c, and the queries with f_b and f_d. Unlike self-attention, we calculate cross-attention between the two modalities. Finally, the fusion of attention weights between the two modalities is multiplied by f_a and f_c, resulting in feature maps f_e and f_g. These fused features are then stacked back onto the main branches for the next stage. To reduce computation complexity, token extraction from branch features can be performed using average pooling to decrease the number of tokens. During the merging process with the branches, upsampling is applied to unify the sizes of the tokens.

Given the input features $X \in \mathbb{R}^{N \times D}$ to the transformer block, where N is the number of tokens in the sequence, and each token is represented by a feature vector of dimension D. We obtain the *Query*, *Key* and *Value* through linear operations:

$$\begin{aligned} Query &= XW_Q, \\ Key &= XW_K, \\ Value &= XW_V \end{aligned} \tag{4}$$

where W_Q, W_K and W_V are weights. It employs the scaled dot-product between *Query* and *Key* to calculate attention weights and then aggregates the values for each *Query*:

$$A = softmax\left(\frac{Query \cdot Key^T}{\sqrt{D}}\right) Value \tag{5}$$

Compute f_a, f_b, f_c and f_d using Eq. (5), and then calculate the output features and f_e and f_g using Eq. (6):

$$f_e = softmax\left(\frac{f_b f_a f_a^T}{\sqrt{D}}\right) f_a, f_g = softmax\left(\frac{f_d f_c f_c^T}{\sqrt{D}}\right) f_c \tag{6}$$

Finally, the fused output features X_{out} are obtained using a non-linear transformation:

$$X_{out} = MLP(f) \pm X \tag{7}$$

where f represents the feature output of each branch, namely, f_a, f_e, f_c and f_g

2.4 Multi-head Pooling Attention Module

Generally, as the network's depth increases, the output features contain higher-level semantic information. Based on this idea, after fusing the branch networks, we introduce

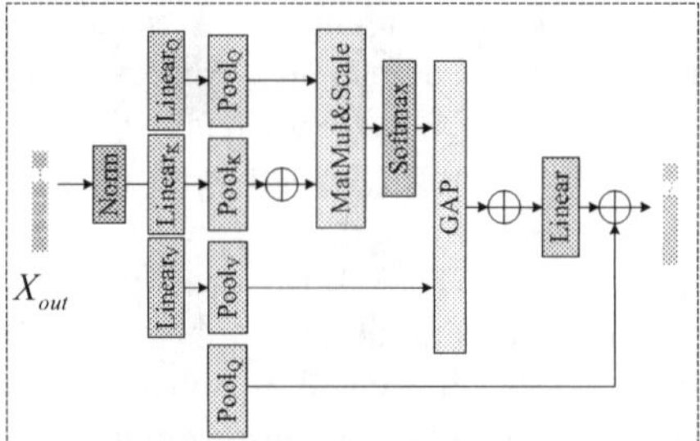

Fig. 3. Illustration of MPA Module

a multi-head pooling module to further learn high-order semantic information. Unlike the original Multi-head Attention (MHA) operator [16], the multi-head pooling module aggregates latent tensor sequences to reduce the length of the input sequences, as shown in Fig. 4. Similar to the MHA, we obtain Query, Key, and Value through linear operations. Then, the MPA incorporates corresponding pooling layers for Query, Key, and Value to further downsample and aggregate the latent tensor sequences, reducing the length of the input sequences involved (Fig. 3).

3 Experiments

3.1 Experimental Configuration

To train the proposed model, we collected data from 200 diagnosed patients with acute ischemic stroke from local hospitals. The inclusion criteria were as follows: (1) patients diagnosed with acute ischemic stroke, (2) recorded time of stroke symptom onset, (3) complete CT perfusion imaging, and (4) availability of complete patient information. The Time Since Stroke (TSS) was calculated by subtracting the time of observing the first stroke symptom from the time of obtaining the first imaging. Based on the TSS range, patients were categorized into two classes: positive if TSS was less than 6 h and negative if TSS was greater than 6 h. All images were preprocessed to a size of $256 \times 256 \times 32$.

We utilized PyTorch for training the model on a single NVIDIA GPU. During the training process, we employed the Adam optimizer and utilized the cross-entropy loss function with an initial learning rate of 10^{-5}. A fixed step-size decay learning strategy was employed, where the step size was set to 15 and γ was set to 0.8, The training was carried out for 30 epoch. Due to the limited amount of available data, we adopted 5-fold cross-validation to train our model.

3.2 Experimental Results and Analysis

To validate the effectiveness of the proposed method in this research, we conducted comparative experiments with other methods. In the comparative study, all methods were tested using the same parameters and experimental strategies to ensure fair comparisons. Based on extensive experimentation, the results of the comparative study are presented in

Table 1 and Fig. 4. From Table 1, it is evident that our model achieves a notable improvement in accuracy compared to other methods on the same dataset. Moreover, for most evaluation metrics, our model consistently outperforms the comparison methods. This demonstrates that our model is superior to these approaches and exhibits commendable performance.

The ROC curves and the corresponding AUC for different methods are illustrated in Fig. 4. Our method achieves an AUC of 81% in the classification task. Clearly, the ROC curve representing our proposed model outperforms those of other models, indicating the superiority of our approach. These findings highlight the robustness of the method used in this research, as it can extract more discriminative features, enabling the network to achieve optimal performance in the classification task.

Table 1. Comparison of results of different methods (%).

Method	Accuracy	Sensitivity	Precision	F1-score	Specificity	Kappa
VGG11	73.55 ± 4.18	86.08 ± 7.60	77.52 ± 3.57	81.17 ± 3.90	47.25 ± 11.76	36.55 ± 11.05
AlexNet	74.22 ± 4.55	85.05 ± 7.18	77.35 ± 3.98	80.93 ± 3.28	52.65 ± 13.55	38.55 ± 10.85
ResNet34	77.50 ± 4.25	91.54 ± 5.57	78.44 ± 4.07	84.43 ± 3.36	49.45 ± 12.96	44.82 ± 11.65
SlowFast [22]	75.98 ± 4.81	85.85 ± 4.75	79.85 ± 4.55	82.05 ± 4.73	57.82 ± 10.07	45.16 ± 10.74
I3D [23]	73.15 ± 4.74	**92.45 ± 7.18**	75.07 ± 5.02	81.99 ± 3.27	34.81 ± 16.99	30.19 ± 14.95
C3D [24]	74.55 ± 2.98	87.29 ± 8.85	78.12 ± 2.89	82.11 ± 2.57	50.88 ± 12.57	40.58 ± 7.18
SSFTTNet [25]	76.05 ± 4.16	89.32 ± 10.00	78.09 ± 3.60	83.00 ± 3.82	49.34 ± 14.17	41.70 ± 8.58
MFNet [26]	74.57 ± 4.39	90.90 ± 6.97	75.79 ± 4.47	81.98 ± 3.93	40.08 ± 16.25	36.71 ± 12.67
CoAtNet [27]	76.05 ± 4.25	91.00 ± 3.25	77.38 ± 4.76	83.51 ± 2.30	46.04 ± 16.20	40.58 ± 13.63
Ours	**80.86** ± 3.99	89.60 ± 5.31	**83.27 ± 4.61**	**86.03 ± 3.56**	**65.93 ± 13.18**	**57.09 ± 8.24**

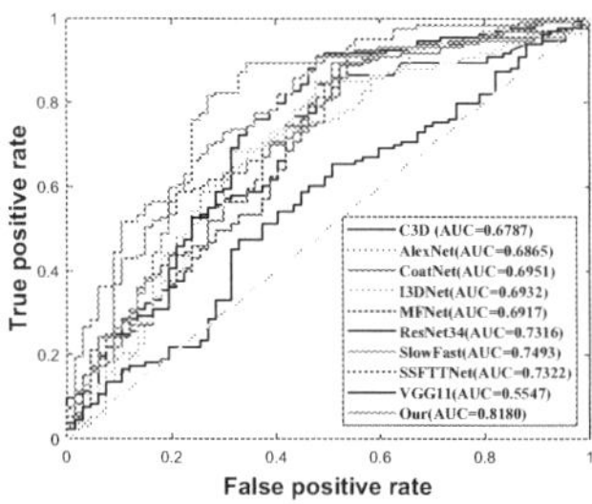

Fig. 4. ROC curve of proposed method and comparison method.

To validate the effectiveness of each module proposed in our method, this section presents a series of ablation experiments by gradually adding these modules to our main network. Table 2 displays the results of the ablation experiments, where different combinations of modules are added to the main network. From the results, it can be observed that each individual module contributes to enhancing the performance of the main network. The inclusion of the CAF module into the main network leads to an improvement in classification accuracy, as it facilitates the fusion of complementary information among different feature maps. Similarly, when adding the MPA module after the main network, it further extracts high-level features, thereby enhancing the overall performance of the model.

In conclusion, the ablation experiments demonstrate that the modules included in the proposed model have a positive impact on its improvement and contribute significantly to its effectiveness.

Table 2. Ablation experiment results.

Module			Accuracy	Sensitivity	Precision	F1-score	Specificity	Kappa
MFE	CAF	MPA						
√			76.05 ± 2.55	89.16 ± 5.90	78.72 ± 3.54	84.05 ± 2.55	53.86 ± 13.28	47.28 ± 14.54
√	√		78.91 ± 2.30	87.44 ± 3.29	81.08 ± 3.89	84.30 ± 1.13	60.43 ± 13.78	54.69 ± 14.95
√		√	78.55 ± 2.68	**89.94 ± 4.15**	80.96 ± 1.55	85.12 ± 2.25	53.63 ± 6.76	54.75 ± 13.94
√	√	√	**80.86 ± 3.99**	89.60 ± 5.31	**83.27 ± 4.61**	**86.03 ± 3.56**	**65.93 ± 13.18**	**57.09 ± 8.24**

4 Conclusion

In this paper, we propose an AIS onset time window detection model based on multi-scale feature extraction and cross attention fusion. Experimental results demonstrate that our model outperforms state-of-the-art methods and provides the best diagnosis performance. In the future, we will strive to explore more deep learning methods for acute ischemic stroke onset time window detection. Additionally, we will investigate further fusion approaches to effectively combine features from perfusion maps, aiming to achieve more clinically meaningful results.

Acknowledgement. This work was supported National Natural Science Foundation of China (Nos. 62201360, 62101338, 61871274, 62271328,and U1902209), National Natural Science Foundation of Guangdong Province (2019A1515111205), Guangdong Basic and Applied Basic Research (2021A1515110746), Shenzhen Key Basic Research Project (KCXFZ20201221173213036,JCYJ20220818095809021,SGDX20201103095 8020-07,JCYJ201908081556188-06,and JCYJ20190808145011259) Capital's Funds for Health Improvement and Research (No. 2022-1-2031), Beijing Hospitals Authority's Ascent Plan (No. DFL20220303), and Beijing Key Specialists in Major Epidemic Prevention and Control.

References

1. Paciaroni, M., Caso, V., Agnelli, G.: The concept of ischemic penumbra in acute stroke and therapeutic opportunities. Eur. Neurol. **61**(6), 321–330 (2009)

2. Hu, H.H., Chu, F.L., Chiang, B.N., Lan, C.F., Sheng, W.Y., Lo, Y.K., et al.: Prevalence of stroke in Taiwan. Stroke **20**(7), 858–863 (1989)
3. Tissue plasminogen activator for acute ischemic stroke. N. Engl. J. Med. **333**(24), 1581-1588 (1995)
4. Ma, H., Campbell, B.C.V., Parsons, M.W., Churilov, L., Levi, C.R., Hsu, C., et al.: Thrombolysis guided by perfusion imaging up to 9 hours after onset of stroke. N. Engl. J. Med. **380**(19), 1795–1803 (2019)
5. Konstas, A., Goldmakher, G., Lee, T.-Y., Lev, M.: Theoretic basis and technical implementations of CT perfusion in acute ischemic stroke, part 1: theoretic basis. Am. J. Neuroradiol. **30**(4), 662–668 (2009)
6. Karthik, R., Menaka, R., Johnson, A., Anand, S.: Neuroimaging and deep learning for brain stroke detection - a review of recent advancements and future prospects. Comput. Methods Programs Biomed. **197**, 105728 (2020)
7. Saver, J.L., Goyal, M., Van der Lugt, A., Menon, B.K., Majoie, C.B., Dippel, D.W., et al.: Time to treatment with endovascular thrombectomy and outcomes from ischemic stroke: a meta-analysis. JAMA **316**(12), 1279–1289 (2016)
8. Govindarajan, P., Soundarapandian, R.K., Gandomi, A.H., Patan, R., Jayaraman, P., Manikandan, R.: Classification of stroke disease using machine learning algorithms. Neural Comput. Appl. **32**(3), 817–828 (2020)
9. Garg, R., Oh, E., Naidech, A., Kording, K., Prabhakaran, S.: Automating ischemic stroke subtype classification using machine learning and natural language processing. J. Stroke Cerebrovasc. Dis. **28**(7), 2045–2051 (2019)
10. Mittermeier, A., et al.: End-to-end deep learning approach for perfusion data: a proof-of-concept study to classify core volume in stroke CT. Diagnostics **12**, 1142 (2022)
11. Dourado, Jr. C.M.J.M., da Silva, S.P.P., da brega, R.V.M., da S. Barros, A.C., Filho, P.P.R., de Albuquerque, V.H.C.: Deep learning IoT system for online stroke detection in skull computed tomography images. Comput. Netw. **152**, 25–39 (2019)
12. Neethi, A.S., Niyas, S., Kannath, S.K., Mathew, J., Anzar, A.M., Rajan, J.: Stroke classification from computed tomography scans using 3D convolutional neural network. Biomed. Signal Process. Control **76**, 103720 (2022)
13. Ho, K.C., Speier, W., Zhang, H., Scalzo, F., El-Saden, S., Arnold, C.W.: A machine learning approach for classifying ischemic stroke onset time from imaging. IEEE Trans. Med. Imaging **38**(7), 1666–1676 (2019)
14. Polson, J.S., Zhang, H., Nael, K., Salamon, N., Yoo, B.Y., El-Saden, S., et al.: Identifying acute ischemic stroke patients within the thrombolytic treatment window using deep learning. J. Neuroimaging **32**(6), 1153–1160 (2022)
15. Chen, C.-F.R., Fan, Q., Panda, R.: Crossvit: cross-attention multi-scale vision transformer for image classification, pp. 357–366 (2021)
16. Vaswani, A., et al.: Attention is all you need. Adv. Neural Inf. Process. Syst. **30** (2017)
17. Dosovitskiy, A., Beyer, L., Kolesnikov, A., Weissenborn, D., Zhai, X., Unterthiner, T., et al.: An image is worth 16x16 words: transformers for image recognition at scale. arXiv preprint arXiv:20101.1929 (2020)
18. Qi, D., Su, L., Song, J., Cui, E., Bharti, T., Sacheti, A.: Imagebert: cross-modal pre-training with large-scale weak-supervised image-text data. arXiv preprint arXiv:20010.7966 (2020)
19. Chen, M., et al. Generative pretraining from pixels. In: International Conference on Machine Learning, pp. 1691–703. PMLR (2020)
20. Sun, C., Myers, A., Vondrick, C., Murphy, K., Schmid, C.: Videobert: a joint model for video and language representation learning. In: Proceedings of the IEEE/CVF International Conference on Computer Vision, pp. 7464–7473 (2019)
21. Zhu, Q., Wang, H., Xu, B., Zhang, Z., Shao, W., Zhang, D.: Multimodal triplet attention network for brain disease diagnosis. IEEE Trans. Med. Imaging **41**(12), 3884–3894 (2022)

22. Feichtenhofer, C., Fan, H., Malik, J., He, K.: Slowfast networks for video recognition. In: Proceedings of the IEEE/CVF International Conference on Computer Vision, pp. 6202–6211 (2019)
23. Carreira, J., Zisserman, A.: Quo vadis, action recognition? a new model and the kinetics dataset. In: Proceedings of the IEEE Conference on Computer Vision and Pattern Recognition, pp. 6299–6308 (2017)
24. Tran, D., Bourdev, L., Fergus, R., Torresani, L., Paluri, M.: Learning spatiotemporal features with 3d convolutional networks. In: Proceedings of the IEEE International Conference on Computer Vision, pp. 4489–4497 (2015)
25. Sun, L., Zhao, G., Zheng, Y., Wu, Z.: Spectral-spatial feature tokenization transformer for hyperspectral image classification. IEEE Trans. Geosci. Remote Sens. **60**, 1–14 (2022)
26. Chen, Y., Kalantidis, Y., Li, J., Yan, S., Feng, J.: Multi-fiber networks for video recognition. In: Proceedings of the European Conference on Computer Vision (ECCV), pp. 352–367 (2018)
27. Dai, Z., Liu, H., Le, Q.V., Tan, M.: Coatnet: marrying convolution and attention for all data sizes. Adv. Neural. Inf. Process. Syst. **34**, 3965–3977 (2021)

Cheap Lunch for Medical Image Segmentation by Fine-Tuning SAM on Few Exemplars

Weijia Feng[1], Lingting Zhu[2], and Lequan Yu[2](✉)

[1] Zhejiang University, Hangzhou, China
22135081@zju.edu.cn
[2] The University of Hong Kong, Hong Kong SAR, China
ltzhu99@connect.hku.hk, lqyu@hku.hk

Abstract. The Segment Anything Model (SAM) has demonstrated remarkable capabilities of scaled-up segmentation models, enabling zero-shot generalization across a variety of domains. By leveraging large-scale foundational models as pre-trained models, it is a natural progression to fine-tune SAM for specific domains to further enhance performances. However, the adoption of foundational models in the medical domain presents a challenge due to the difficulty and expense of labeling sufficient data for adaptation within hospital systems. In this paper, we introduce an efficient and practical approach for fine-tuning SAM using a limited number of exemplars, making it suitable for such scenarios. Our approach combines two established techniques from the literature: an exemplar-guided synthesis module and the widely recognized Low-Rank Adaptation (LoRA) fine-tuning strategy, serving as data-level and model-level attempts respectively. Interestingly, our empirical findings suggest that SAM can be effectively aligned within the medical domain even with few labeled data. We validate our approach through experiments on brain tumor segmentation (BraTS) and multi-organ CT segmentation (Synapse). The comprehensive results underscore the feasibility and effectiveness of such an approach, paving the way for the practical application of SAM in the medical domain.

Keywords: Medical Image Segmentation · Foundation Models · Segment Anything Model (SAM) · Few Exemplars

1 Introduction

Nowadays, foundation models [3] have revolutionized the AI community, demonstrating immense potential to solve tasks within an integrated framework and achieve remarkable zero-shot and few-shot performances [4,8]. The Segment Anything Model (SAM) [14], a promptable model trained on over 1 billion masks and 11 million images, makes an attempt to build a foundation model for segmentation. SAM has shown impressive zero-shot segmentation ability on new

U. Baid et al. (Eds.): BrainLes 2023/SWITCH 2023, LNCS 14668, pp. 13–22, 2024.
https://doi.org/10.1007/978-3-031-76160-7_2

data across different distributions and tasks. However, SAM's performance has been found to be limited in certain domains, such as medical images segmentation [7,12,21], low-level structural segmentation [7], and intricate objection segmentation [13]. To address these limitations, researchers have sought to enhance the performance of pre-trained models across domains by fine-tuning SAM or externally designed components [7,13,16,21]. As a result, fine-tuning SAM with medical images could be more feasible and promising to facilitate segmentation tasks in real clinical applications [21].

Despite these advancements, the adoption of medical segmentation in real hospitals remains challenging due to the need for large curated datasets. Fine-tuning SAM on labeled images of specific instruments is also required to align model's understanding of the domain scope within the hospital. This introduces a time-consuming, labor-intensive, and expensive process of data labeling [20]. Consequently, there is growing interest in developing effective methods to leverage limited annotated data for training deep learning models [5,9,20].

Among the various attempts to utilize small sets of labeled data, we consider exemplar-based learning an intriguing approach. This scenario, which involves using a single expert-annotated image that covers all parts of the whole organ category set [9], can significantly reduce the labeling expenses in hospital systems. This raises the question: **Can we fine-tune foundation models (SAM) on few exemplars to achieve significant improvements in medical image segmentation?**

In this paper, we integrate two well-established techniques from the literature to serve as the data-level and model-level attempts. On the data-level, we employ the exemplar-guided synthesis module in [9] to generate a synthetic training dataset through geometric and intensity transformation. On the model-level, our fine-tuning strategy is based on the widely recognized Low-Rank Adaptation (LoRA) [11] and specifically, we adhere to the basic architecture outlined in [21]. Notably, we configure the ViT-Base image encoder and update a total of 6.32 million parameters. Unlike many works relying on A100 40/80G GPUs, all of our experiments are executable on more accessible GPUs such as the 3090 24G GPUs.

We assess the effectiveness of our approach on two medical image segmentation tasks: brain tumor segmentation (BraTS 2018 [1,2,17]) and multi-organ CT segmentation (Synapse[1]). Extensive results suggest that fine-tuning SAM on a few exemplars can strike a balance between accuracy and annotation labor, offering a cost-effective solution for medical image segmentation. In summary, our contributions are twofold: (1) We introduce the attempt of fine-tuning the foundation segmentation model SAM with few exemplars for medical image segmentation. (2) We present comprehensive results on two datasets from different sub-domains, using only 1% labeled data, demonstrating the feasibility of this cost-effective solution.

[1] https://www.synapse.org/#!Synapse:syn3193805/wiki/217789.

2 Methods

2.1 Synthesized Dataset Based on Exemplars

Given limited labeled exemplars, to generate substituted training dataset comprising of more data samples, we adopt the exemplar-based synthesis module proposed in [9] to create more synthesized data. For each organ or tumor cropped from exemplars, we apply geometric and intensity transformations including blur, intensity variation, scale, flip and rotation to it before pasting it onto similarly transformed background images. Background images are chosen from slices in training volumes without organs or tumors. Due to the different numbers of the segmentation labels in the two datasets, we use different processes for BraTS 2018 (tumor) and Synapse (multi-organ). The processes can be depicted by the following equations.

For the BraTS 2018, the generating of synthesized images can be described by

$$I_s = \mathcal{T}(I_e \otimes Y_e) \quad if \quad \mathcal{T}(I_e \otimes Y_e) > 0 \quad else \quad \mathcal{T}(I_b), \tag{1}$$

where $\mathcal{T}$ denotes the transformation, I_s, I_b, I_e, Y_e indicate the synthesized image, background image, exemplar image and exemplar label respectively. The 0 in the equation refers to the value of background pixels. The label of synthesized images can be extracted naturally from above operations.

Since exemplars from the Synapse contain multiple organs, we follow the category-wise manner in [9]. We first apply the above equation to each organ and then merge these organs into the same background image after transformation, which can be described as follows:

$$O_s^k = \mathcal{T}(I_e \otimes Y_e^k), \tag{2}$$

$$I_s = Merge(O_s^1, ..., O_s^K) \quad if \quad Merge(O_s^1, ..., O_s^K) > 0 \quad else \quad \mathcal{T}(I_b), \tag{3}$$

where Y_e^k and O_s^k refer to the label and the transformed image of the k-th organ respectively. The k is in $\{1, ..., K\}$ and K is the total classes. When pasting the synthesized organs onto the background image, we kept the position of the synthesized organs on the background image roughly consistent with their position in the exemplar.

2.2 Fine-Tuning SAM

Low-Rank Adaptation (LoRA [11]) is originally proposed as a fine-tune strategy that applies low rank decomposition matrices for Transformer [19] based large language model. The basic idea can be summarized as updating the pre-trained weight matrix with a low-rank decomposed bypass matrix. The bypass matrix can be treated as the multiplication of two matrices $A \in \mathbb{R}^{r \times C_{in}}$ and $B \in \mathbb{R}^{C_{out} \times r}$ with the low-rank constraint, *i.e.*, $r \ll \min(C_{in}, C_{out})$. As a result, given a projection layer $W \in \mathbb{R}^{C_{out} \times C_{in}}$, the updated projection is described as $\hat{W} = W + \Delta W = W + BA$.

Following the key design in LoRA, the basic operations adopting LoRA in computer vision tasks may involve firstly freezing all parameters in the pre-trained model and then applying trainable bypass matrices as projection layers for transformer blocks. In practice, we follow the basic backbone in SAMed [21] of using LoRA to fine-tune SAM on medical images. Different from SAMed, we investigate point-based prompting in SAM and fine-tune the mask decoder with the point-based prompt embedding. SAMed utilizes LoRA in the query and value projection layers and it is optional to fine-tune all the parameters or apply LoRA to the lightweight mask decoder of SAM. In our implementation, we observe that applying LoRA to the mask decoder achieves better performance in our setting. In order to incorporate point prompts for training all classes simultaneously, we randomly select one class and randomly sample a point from pixels belong to this class during training. In the end, the mask decoder outputs two classes including a background class and the target class. We apply LoRA to both the image encoder and the mask decoder with rank $r = 4$, and there are only 6.32M trainable parameters, which are 1.77% of SAM that using ViT-B as image encoder. Our fine-tune strategy only needs to train a small number of parameters and serve as a cost-effective solution.

3 Experiments

3.1 Datasets

We conduct experiments on two medical datasets including the BraTS 2018 [1,2, 17] and the Synapse Dataset. BraTS 2018 contains 285 MRI scans in the original training split, and we randomly split those scans into 80% for training and the remaining 20% for testing. The final train set contains 228 scans with a total of 38340 slices, of which 14662 have tumors with no fewer than 10 pixels. For this dataset, we use the FLAIR modality to segment the whole tumor like these papers [10,16]. For each image in BraTS, we normalize the pixel values to the range [0, 1] using min-max normalization. The Synapse dataset is from MICCAI 2015 Multi-Atlas Abdomen Labeling Challenge, consisting of 30 abdominal CT scans. Following division settings in TransUNet [6], 30 cases in Synapse are divided into 18 training cases and 12 testing cases with eight organs. 18 training cases contain 2212 axial slices in total. All Images in Synapse are clipped to [-125, 275] before min-max normalized into [0, 1]. Dice Similarity Score (DSC) and 95% Hausdorff Distance (HD95) are used as the evaluation metrics.

3.2 Exemplar Selection

Due to the different characteristics of the two datasets, we select exemplars with different strategies. For the BraTS 2018 dataset, since our segmentation target is the whole tumor solely, we randomly select exemplars from all training images that having tumors with a portions of 0.5%, 1% and 3% respectively. For the Synapse dataset, each slice has a different number of organs. We select 9, 18 and 36 exemplars that have most organs in training volumes since the imbalanced organ distribution can lead to poor segmentation results for some organs. Specifically, for the 9 exemplars case, we select 9 from all training volumes, and then choose one image with the most organs from each of the selected volume as an exemplar. We select one and two images from each training volume for the 18 and 36 exemplars cases respectively.

3.3 Implementation Details

For the substitute training dataset synthesis, we ensure that for all different exemplar numbers, the synthesized datasets are of the same size, *i.e.*, 4500 for the BraTS 2018 and 1800 for the the Synapse Dataset. Cross entropy loss and dice loss are adopted to optimize trainable parameters. The overall loss function can be written as $L = \lambda_1 L_{CE} + \lambda_2 L_{Dice}$, where λ_1 is set to 1 and λ_2 is set to 0.8 empirically. We use the AdamW [15] optimizer with an initial learning rate of $\alpha = 0.001$. Warm up and exponential decay are adopted to schedule the learning rate. All experiments are run on two NVIDIA GeForce RTX 3090 GPUs (Fig. 1).

Table 1. Quantitative comparison on the BraTS 2018.

Methods	Exemplar Nums	DSC ↑	HD ↓
SAM (Zero-Shot)	–	45.29	54.74
SAMed (w/ Data Synthesis)	75 (0.5%)	82.80	28.03
	150 (1%)	82.50	43.99
	450 (3%)	85.53	17.56
	Total Nums	85.52	31.13
Ours	75 (0.5%)	82.78	14.92
	150 (1%)	83.4	10.03
	450 (3%)	83.07	16.94
Full Set (Pseudo Upper Bound)	Total Nums	85.28	7.91

Table 2. Quantitative comparison on the Synapse multi-organ CT dataset.

Methods	Exemplar Nums	DSC ↑	HD ↓	Aorta	Gallbladder	Kidney(L)	Kidney(R)	Liver	Pancreas	Spleen	Stomach
SAM	–	74.54	40.90	88.74	40.55	87.11	82.60	88.63	53.77	83.79	71.14
Att-UNet [18]	Total Nums	77.77	36.02	89.55	68.88	77.98	71.11	93.57	58.04	87.30	75.75
SAMed	9 (one per two volumes)	43.82	96.21	40.50	34.20	44.35	46.10	81.32	23.43	43.86	36.78
	18 (one per volume)	55.26	75.02	45.28	50.70	58.75	62.53	87.58	31.07	72.82	33.32
	36 (one per volume)	66.96	44.69	63.75	58.17	72.97	68.96	90.67	40.38	80.40	60.35
	Total Nums	81.88	20.64	87.77	69.11	80.45	79.95	94.80	72.17	88.72	82.06
Ours	1 (one exemplar)	75.91	21.75	84.46	49.56	83.74	84.92	88.05	56.43	89.28	70.80
	9 (one per two volumes)	79.08	21.62	88.75	55.76	88.35	84.11	89.76	61.26	91.27	73.41
	18 (one per volume)	83.04	16.84	89.18	71.33	89.20	86.46	92.55	64.20	90.52	80.84
	36 (two per volume)	84.23	11.86	88.31	69.91	90.43	88.57	94.82	65.17	91.36	85.24
Full Set	Total Nums	85.95	8.97	91.52	64.42	92.49	91.56	96.06	66.49	94.39	90.66

3.4 Results

Our main results are shown in Table 1 and Table 2. We compare our results on different exemplar numbers with the results tested on SAM (zero-shot), SAMed, and Full Set for both datasets, where Full Set represents the results of our model on the full training dataset without synthesized data. Notably, the SAM that we use in the test stage is configured with ViT-H (Huge), which is based on the huge ViT encoder that yields the best performance, while the others are configured with ViT-B (Base). For SAM, Ours, and Full Set, we provide one point prompt for each class (except the background class) of each slice in testing. These points are selected from those furthest from the margin of test classes. For SAMed, we use the synthesized dataset as Ours and use the default prompt embedding in [21] which does not require point prompt and investigates autonomous segmentation. Total Nums in the Exemplar Nums column of all tables means using all images in train sets without synthesized data. Especially, for the Full Set, since we use the full set training set which is not synthesized and we keep the same training pipeline as ours, this method can be treated as the pseudo upper bound. The HD in all table headers represents the HD95.

Table 1 shows the performance of SAM, SAMed, Ours, and Full Set on the BraTS. The results tested directly with SAM are poor, indicating the SAM

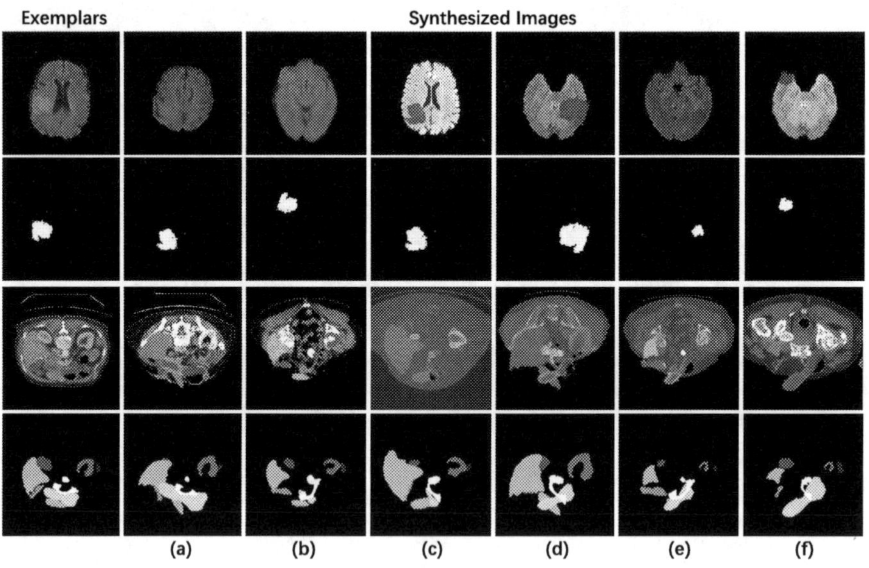

Fig. 1. Synthesized data samples. The images are shown in the 1-st and 3-rd rows, while their corresponding labels are presented in the 2-nd and 4-th rows. The first column shows the exemplars, and the subsequent columns present several synthesized data samples. Geometric and intensity transformations including blur, intensity variation, scale, flip and rotation are applied during data synthesis process. The transformed tumor or organs are pasted onto randomly selected background images.

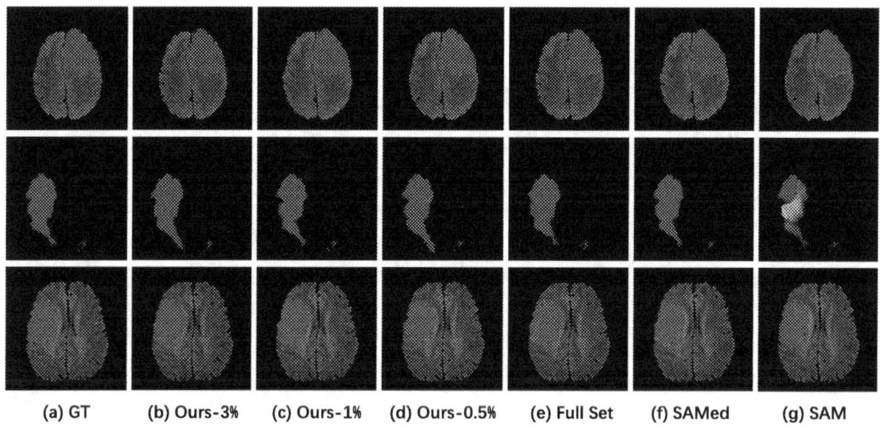

Fig. 2. The qualitative comparisons on the BraTS 2018.

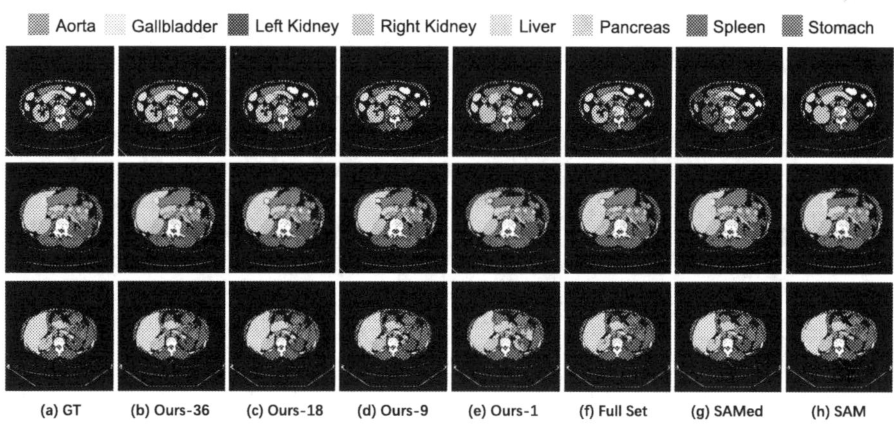

Fig. 3. The qualitative comparisons on the Synapse multi-organ CT dataset.

may fail to segment anything in the medical domain. All fine-tuned models achieve much better performances. Trained on the synthesized dataset based on 0.5% of the total data, SAMed and Ours achieve rather good test results. Our model outperforms SAMed on HD95 slightly in all test cases. Figure 2 gives the qualitative comparison results on the BraTS 2018.

Table 2 shows the results of SAM, Att-UNet, SAMed, Ours, and Full Set on the Synapse. The SAM yields decent results when tested directly on this dataset while SAMed performs poorly when trained on synthesized dataset generated by few exemplars. In contrast, Ours achieves rather good segmentation results with the synthesized dataset using few exemplars. The results of Ours (ViT-B) trained on the dataset generated from only one exemplar is slightly better than SAM (ViT-H) zero-shot performance. When the number of exemplars comes to 18, the DSC and HD95 in the results are better than those tested on SAM

Table 3. Quantitative comparison between w/o and w/ data synthesis on the BraTS.

Methods	Exemplar Nums	DSC ↑	HD ↓
w/o Data Synthesis	75 (0.5%)	68.14	17.85
	150 (1%)	81.76	18.43
	450 (3%)	81.02	11.14
w/ Data Synthesis	75 (0.5%)	82.78	14.92
	150 (1%)	83.4	10.03
	450 (3%)	83.07	16.94

Table 4. Quantitative comparison between w/o and w/ data synthesis on the Synapse.

Methods	Exemplar Nums	DSC ↑	HD ↓	Aorta	Gallbladder	Kidney(L)	Kidney(R)	Liver	Pancreas	Spleen	Stomach
w/o Data Synthesis	9 (one per two volumes)	78.36	24.11	85.67	52.14	87.17	85.64	86.46	64.11	88.72	76.99
	18 (one per volume)	79.01	20.37	86.69	52.02	87.68	86.00	88.20	63.56	90.44	77.46
	36 (three per volume)	80.82	18.22	89.60	50.51	87.36	87.23	92.29	65.94	92.44	81.20
w/ Data Synthesis	9 (one per two volumes)	79.08	21.62	88.75	55.76	88.35	84.11	89.76	61.26	91.27	73.41
	18 (one per volume)	83.04	16.84	89.18	71.33	89.20	86.46	92.55	64.20	90.52	80.84
	36 (three per volume)	84.23	11.86	88.31	69.91	90.43	88.57	94.82	65.17	91.36	85.24

by 8.5% and 24.06 respectively. The qualitative comparison results are given in Fig. 3.

Comparing the results on two datasets, we find that point prompts play a more important role in the multi-organ segmentation. We believe that it is because the task of multi-organ segmentation is much harder than the whole tumor segmentation. Though our method is not an automatic solution to medical image segmentation, we attempt to investigate the point prompt setting and demonstrate that our method achieves impressive result with few exemplars. Especially for datasets lacking annotations, our method provides a cost-effective solution to achieve satisfactory segmentation results.

3.5 Ablation Studies

Furthermore, we compare the performances of training on synthesized datasets with those of training on simply exemplars. The results are displayed in Table 3 and Table 4. We can see that for both datasets, training on the generated dataset yields better results than training simply with exemplars. This ablation study indicates that on the one hand, a small portion of training data can train the model fairly well, demonstrating SAM has strong learning ability on segmentation. On the other hand, using synthesized data besides exemplars brings obvious improvement to the model performance, shows that exemplar-based data synthesis plays a vital role in improving model performances. The test results using random point prompts are given in Table 5 amd Table 6.

Table 5. Quantitative results with random point prompts on the BraTS.

Methods	Exemplar Nums	DSC ↑	HD ↓
SAM	–	44.93	55.36
[1]*Ours	75 (0.5%)	82.88	14.49
	150 (1%)	83.50	14.78
	450 (3%)	83.04	14.78
Full Set	Total Nums	85.28	7.92

Table 6. Quantitative results with random point prompts on the Synapse.

Methods	Exemplar Nums	DSC ↑	HD ↓	Aorta	Gallbladder	Kidney(L)	Kidney(R)	Liver	Pancreas	Spleen	Stomach
SAM	–	74.49	41.15	88.73	40.58	87.11	82.55	88.59	53.67	83.64	71.06
[1]*Ours	1 (one exemplar)	72.88	25.36	82.32	43.64	83.66	83.55	84.46	50.72	89.46	50.72
	9 (one per two volumes)	76.83	16.05	88.40	52.45	87.59	82.84	87.15	57.58	88.97	69.64
	18 (one per volume)	78.53	26.74	88.03	53.61	88.50	86.27	89.08	59.08	87.64	76.06
	36 (two per volume)	81.25	17.20	88.23	58.63	90.28	87.70	92.50	60.15	90.49	82.70
Full Set	Total Nums	85.06	12.43	90.59	60.68	91.54	90.07	94.75	62.13	94.08	88.64

4 Conclusion

In this paper, we explore the potential of fine-tuning the Segment Anything Model with few exemplars for medical image segmentation. Our approach, which integrates an exemplar-guided synthesis module and the low-rank-based fine-tuning strategy as the data-level and the model-level attempts, has demonstrated promising results in brain tumor segmentation and multi-organ CT segmentation tasks. The experimental results indicate the feasibility of achieving a balance between accuracy and annotation labor, thereby offering a cost-effective solution for medical image segmentation. Looking ahead, we believe that the effective utilization of limited labeled data remains an open problem, particularly in the current era where foundational models present both opportunities and challenges. Furthermore, the integration of a small number of labeled exemplars with a large amount of unlabeled data is an area that deserves further investigation. We hope our attempts present an important initial step towards the practical application of pre-trained models in the medical domain.

Acknowledgement. The work described in this paper was partially supported by grants from the National Natural Science Fund (62201483) and the Research Grants Council of the Hong Kong Special Administrative Region, China (T45-401/22-N).

References

1. Bakas, S., et al.: Advancing the cancer genome atlas glioma MRI collections with expert segmentation labels and radiomic features. Sci. Data **4**(1), 1–13 (2017)
2. Bakas, S., et al.: Identifying the best machine learning algorithms for brain tumor segmentation, progression assessment, and overall survival prediction in the brats challenge. arXiv preprint arXiv:1811.02629 (2018)
3. Bommasani, R., et al.: On the opportunities and risks of foundation models. arXiv preprint arXiv:2108.07258 (2021)
4. Brown, T., et al.: Language models are few-shot learners. Adv. Neural. Inf. Process. Syst. **33**, 1877–1901 (2020)
5. Chaitanya, K., Erdil, E., Karani, N., Konukoglu, E.: Contrastive learning of global and local features for medical image segmentation with limited annotations. Adv. Neural. Inf. Process. Syst. **33**, 12546–12558 (2020)
6. Chen, J., et al.: Transunet: transformers make strong encoders for medical image segmentation. arXiv preprint arXiv:2102.04306 (2021)
7. Chen, T., et al.: Sam fails to segment anything?–sam-adapter: adapting sam in underperformed scenes: camouflage, shadow, and more. arXiv preprint arXiv:2304.09148 (2023)
8. Chowdhery, A., et al.: Palm: scaling language modeling with pathways. arXiv preprint arXiv:2204.02311 (2022)
9. En, Q., Guo, Y.: Exemplar learning for medical image segmentation. arXiv preprint arXiv:2204.01713 (2022)
10. Ghorbel, A., Aldahdooh, A., Albarqouni, S., Hamidouche, W.: Transformer based models for unsupervised anomaly segmentation in brain mr images. arXiv preprint arXiv:2207.02059 (2022)
11. Hu, E.J., et al.: Lora: low-rank adaptation of large language models. arXiv preprint arXiv:2106.09685 (2021)
12. Huang, Y., et al.: Segment anything model for medical images? arXiv preprint arXiv:2304.14660 (2023)
13. Ke, L., et al.: Segment anything in high quality. arXiv preprint arXiv:2306.01567 (2023)
14. Kirillov, A., et al.: Segment anything. arXiv preprint arXiv:2304.02643 (2023)
15. Loshchilov, I., Hutter, F.: Decoupled weight decay regularization. arXiv preprint arXiv:1711.05101 (2017)
16. Ma, J., He, Y., Li, F., Han, L., Chenyu, Y., Wang, B.: Segment anything in medical images. arXiv preprint arXiv:2304.12306 (2023)
17. Menze, B.H., et al.: The multimodal brain tumor image segmentation benchmark (brats). IEEE Trans. Med. Imaging **34**(10), 1993–2024 (2014)
18. Oktay, O., et al.: Attention u-net: learning where to look for the pancreas. arXiv preprint arXiv:1804.03999 (2018)
19. Vaswani, A., et al.: Attention is all you need. Adv. Neural Inf. Process. Syst. **30** (2017)
20. Wang, S., et al.: Annotation-efficient deep learning for automatic medical image segmentation. Nat. Commun. **12**(1), 5915 (2021)
21. Zhang, K., Liu, D.: Customized segment anything model for medical image segmentation. arXiv preprint arXiv:2304.13785 (2023)

BeSt-LeS: Benchmarking Stroke Lesion Segmentation using Deep Supervision

Prantik Deb(✉), Lalith Bharadwaj Baru, Kamalaker Dadi, and Bapi Raju S

Brain Cognitive Computation Lab, Cognitive Science, IIIT, Hyderabad, Hyderabad 500032, India

prantik.deb@ihub-data.iiit.ac.in, lalith.baru@research.iiit.ac.in

Abstract. Brain stroke has become a significant burden on global health and thus we need remedies and prevention strategies to overcome this challenge. For this, the immediate identification of stroke and risk stratification is the primary task for clinicians. To aid expert clinicians, automated segmentation models are crucial. In this work, we consider the publicly available dataset ATLAS v2.0 to benchmark various end-to-end supervised U-Net style models. Specifically, we have benchmarked models on both 2D and 3D brain images and evaluated them using standard metrics. We have achieved the highest Dice score of 0.583 on the 2D transformer-based model and 0.504 on the 3D residual U-Net respectively. We have conducted the Wilcoxon test for 3D models to correlate the relationship between predicted and actual stroke volume. For reproducibility, the code and model weights are made publicly available: link.

Keywords: Stroke Lesion Segmentation · T1 Weighted MRI · Deep Supervision · ATLAS v2.0 · Deep Learning

1 Introduction

Brain stroke has become a significant burden on global health with increasing prevalence in low- and middle-income countries. Therefore there is an urgent need for targeted prevention strategies and improved healthcare infrastructure to address this growing public health challenge [19], [21]. Given brain Magnetic Resonance (MR) images on stroke populations, localizing and detecting the lesions is crucial for clinicians. However, the automation of the localization process has achieved significant reach [5] with novel machine-learning models that can aid clinicians. To fuel these models, we need datasets that could automatically segment to the level of expertise and doing so, it could ease the clinician's task.

In this context, ATLAS (Anatomical Tracings of Lesions After Stroke) v1.2 dataset made progress by creating 304 T1-weighted MRI samples collected from 11 cohorts. This ATLAS v1.2 [23] was released in 2018 and of which, 229 standardized subjects were available with T1-weighted MRI image and its corresponding lesion mask. Later in 2022, ATLAS v2.0 [24] was released and it has 1217 T1-weighted MRI samples collected from 44 cohorts of which 655 samples

U. Baid et al. (Eds.): BrainLes 2023/SWITCH 2023, LNCS 14668, pp. 23–35, 2024.
https://doi.org/10.1007/978-3-031-76160-7_3

Table 1. The table summarizes the glimpse of 2D and 3D U-Net variants whether they were implemented on the ATLAS v1.2 and v2.0 T1 MR images denoted as Yes or No. The implementation of 2D models on ATLAS v2.0 is sparse.

2D Models	ATLAS v1.2	ATLAS v2.0
U-Net	Yes [40] [29] [43] [41] [32]	No
Residual U-Net	Yes [40] [29] [32]	No
Attention U-Net	Yes [32]	No
Transformer Based	Yes [38]	No
3D Models	**ATLAS v1.2**	**ATLAS v2.0**
U-Net	Yes [43] [41] [27]	Yes [35] [16]
Residual U-Net	Yes [33]	Yes [16]
Attention U-Net	No	No
Transformer Based	No	No

mask were availed to the public. In specific, there was an extra margin of 426 samples from version 1.2 to 2.0.

There were numerous impressive models that performed well on ATLAS v1.2. Whereas, ATLAS v2.0 was released recently and therefore, there is quite less progress. Therefore, we outpace and benchmark ATLAS v2.0 on various standard U-Net style architectures for both 2D and 3D brain images.

In Table 1, ATLAS v1.2 was applied using distinct U-Net architectures for 2D modality but, there isn't any model to date that has been implemented on ATLAS v2.0. Similarly, in the case of 3D modality, Table 1 illustrates there are few implementations for ATLAS v2.0 using nnU-Net as their underlying framework [17]. Thus, we contribute by analyzing the ATLAS v2.0 dataset for both 2D and 3D modality. A brief description of each of the models is detailed in the supplementary material.

2 Contributions of this Work

1. To the best of our knowledge, ours is the first attempt to benchmark the standard segmentation models *i.e.* both convolution and transformers-based architectures on the ATLAS v2.0 dataset.
2. We have also conducted experiments for both 2D and 3D-based models. We report our highest dice score of 0.58 on the 2D transformer-based model. Also, we have achieved a 0.504 dice score on the 3D residual U-Net.
3. Finally, we conduct the Wilcoxon test on 3D models and compare the relationship between predicted and actual stroke volume.

3 Data and Models

This section briefly discusses the dataset and methods considered for analysis. The organization is as follows: First, we introduce the dataset and the training strategy implied. Next, we detail the significance of various U-Net style models.

3.1 Dataset

The ATLAS (Anatomical Tracings of Lesions After Stroke) data consists of T1-weighted MRI images of subjects having lesions due to stroke. This data has two versions, ATLAS v1.2 [23], and ATLAS v2.0 [24], respectively. For our analysis, we solely conduct our experiments on ATLAS v2.0 dataset [24], which is publicly available[1]. The samples in this data (ATLAS v2.0) were collected from 44 diverse cohorts with a total sample size of 1271. From these 1271 samples, only 655 samples consist of image-to-mask pairs dedicated to training the models. Another 300 samples are treated as hidden-set and do not reveal the masks of T1-weighted MRI images[2].

Table 2. The below table describes the train validation and test proportions divided for training supervised 2D U-Net style architectures. The number of samples below represents the number of subjects. The slices are unevenly divided based on the volume of the T1-weighted MRI and the axial plane is considered while cropping each slice.

Split	%	Samples	Slices
Train	60	393	15394
Validation	20	131	4666
Test	20	131	5452

Table 3. In the below tabular data, the train validation and test proportions are divided for training supervised 3D U-Net style architectures. The number of samples below represents the number of subjects.

Split	%	Samples
Train	60	393
Validation	20	131
Test	20	131

While analyzing ATLAS v2.0 we conduct experiments both on 2D and 3D modality. As masks for the original test set are inaccessible we divide the training samples (655) into train validation and test proportions. For 3D modality, the data can be directly fed to the model. But for 2D modality, each subject's 3D T1-weighted MRI images are to be cropped into slices along the z-axis (axial) and then given as input to 2D U-Net style architectures. For both the modalities the Z-score Normalization are performed as a pre-processing step [2]. The information regarding train, test, and validation sets are elucidated in Table 2 and 3. For the 2D dataset, the discrepancy between the validation and the test is due to a rejection of 0.1% lesions in the given 2D slice. Specifically, wherever the slices and their respective mask pairs were rejected were not included in the study. Now, this data is to be processed using various segmentation architectures to segment the lesion in the T1-weighted MRI images in the protocol mentioned in Table 2 and 3.

[1] The dataset can be found at: link.

[2] Additional information such as lesion numbers, cortical location, and severity of stroke for each subject can be found in the original paper [24].

3.2 U-Net Style Architectures

The delineation of a specific organ or certain tissue site or cell nuclei from given medical images is one of the crucial tasks in medical image analysis. Various deterministic algorithms were developed to automate this process, some of which are random walks [14] and SLIC [1]. But later with the aid of deep learning, more sophisticated and *learnable* methods were developed [12]. Later, Ronneberger *et al.* [31] proposed U-Net architecture from which the field of medical image segmentation caught its attention as U-Net was fast, modulable, and robust. Later there were many methods that were crafted using the U-Net style as the underlying framework. Thus, we study and benchmark some of the fundamental U-Net style architectures that achieved significant results in the field of medical image segmentation.

U-Net: This was the first deep learning architecture that superseded the existing models with large margins both computationally and performance-wise. This architecture, thus, was made as a baseline for many medical segmentation tasks [31]. Soon after the U-Net, the architecture was modified to learn volumetric data using 3D convolutions [11] with sparse annotations. The architecture is very similar to that of 2D U-Net except that, 3D can process volumetric information using 3D convolutions and it is depicted in the last row of Fig. 1.

The architecture is quite intuitive, as features are downsampled using pooling layers to a latent space or base and later upsampled to reconstruct the desired mask image. This latent space is perceived to preserve the crucial features, while the skip-connections (these are denoted as $(\cdots)$) aid the reconstruction by guiding to map of the structural information. In the Fig. 1, you can see each blue circle represents a series of convolution layers, and the red arrow ($\rightarrow$) indicates that an image of size $h \times w$ is downsampled (pooled) to $\frac{h}{2} \times \frac{w}{2}$. The downsampling operation is quadruply performed to get to the latent space. Now, from this latent space, the acquired features are upsampled quadruply (indicated with a green arrow ($\rightarrow$)) to produce the desired segmentation.

Residual U-Net: He *et al.* [15] proved that residual connections tend to provide refined representations for downstream tasks with less computation and better performance. In this regard, Zhang *et al.* [42] proposed a U-Net architecture with residual connections for extracting road patterns from aerial imagery. This later was implied in the domain of medical images by Alom *et al.* [3] with additional memory components. Later, the residual connections were implied between a series of 3D convolutions to produce volumetric segmentation [7,18,39]. The architecture is very similar to that of 2D residual U-Net except that, 3D can produce volumetric masks from 3D medical data, and the pictorial interpretations are illustrated in the last row of Fig. 1.

The current Residual U-Net style was inspired by Zhang *et al.* [42]. In U-Net, before downsampling at each step, there are a series of convolutions with residual connections, which are represented by an orange circle. The rest, upsampling ($\rightarrow$) and downsampling ($\rightarrow$) operations, are similar to that of traditional U-Net.

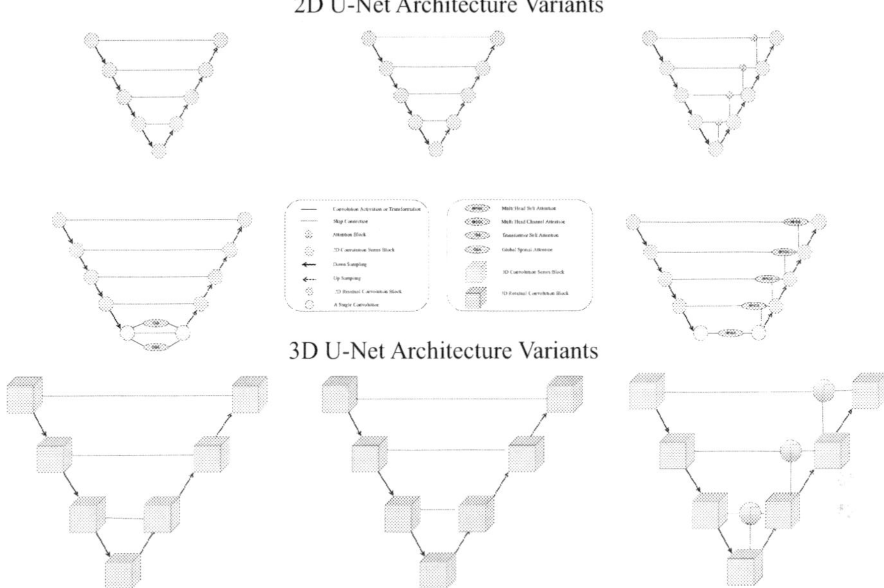

Fig. 1. The figure illustrates various U-Net style architectures. (First row) shows a diagrammatic view of the convolution-based Transformer models and (bottom row) shows two novel transformer-based U-Net architectures. We detailed all the symbols and signs used in the legend block. (Color figure online)

Attention U-Net: The fundamental concept of *attention* was formulated by Bahdanau *et al.* [4]. Later Oktay *et al.* [26] applied this mechanism as '*Attention Gate*' (AG), which improved segmentation with detailed localization of multiple organs.

In this architecture, the core component is the attention gate which aids the U-Net in segmenting desired lesions. The architecture style in downsampling is similar to U-Net, i.e., the image is quadruply downsampled (⟶ ×4) to obtain the latent space. In traditional U-Net, upsampling (⇠) is achieved using transpose convolutions, and additional representations are aggregated from the skip connections. But in Attention U-Net, the representations from the previous layers and from skip connections are aggregated using AG, and now these features are concatenated with the upsampled (⇠) features. Thus, they form cascaded connections resulting in better segmentation. Similarly, this attention gate is applied to 3D convolutions to get volumetric attention [25,36].

TransAttn U-Net: This architecture was designed by Chen *et al.* [10] in which they propose SAA: Self-Aware Attention, which is an amalgamation of multi-level and multi-scale guided attention mechanisms. In specific, after downsampling features to the embedding space, they perform two attention mechanisms which are Transformer Self-Attention ($\mathcal{F}_{TSA}$) and Global Spatial Atten-

Table 4. The below table illustrates the performance of variants of 2D U-Net architectures. The first three models are pure convolution-based architectures and the remaining two are hybrid networks with convolutions and transformer components. The evaluation criteria implied is the same as Table 2; We report the performance of the model for the test set.

Method	Performance Metrics (2D Data)			
	Dice Score	IoU Score	Precision	Recall
U-Net [31]	0.417	0.337	0.580	0.360
Residual U-Net [42]	0.456	0.375	0.592	0.420
Attention U-Net [26]	0.487	0.396	0.636	0.439
TransAttn U-Net [10]	0.572	0.477	**0.660**	0.565
U-Net Transformer [28]	**0.583**	**0.475**	0.659	**0.591**

tion ($\mathcal{F}_{GSA}$). Now, these features are combined into a single convolution block, and with each step of upsampling, the previous layer features are attached as skip connections using *Bi-linear Upsampling* (refer Fig. 1). The significance of each attention mechanism is elucidated below.

Suppose our image is represented as $X \in \mathbb{R}^{t \times h \times w}$, where t, h, w are time-steps (channels), height, and width of the given image, respectively. The image is passed to the encoder, and the downsampled representation is denoted by $\mathcal{F}^t_{base} \in \mathbb{R}^{t \times (h \times w)}$. Now, to achieve GSA,

$$\mathcal{F}_{GSA}(M, N, W)_i = \sum_{k=1}^{h \times w} (W_k \mathcal{A}_{i,j}) \tag{1}$$

where, $N \in \mathbb{R}^{t' \times (h \times w)}$ and $M \in \mathbb{R}^{(h \times w) \times t'}$. Also the $\mathcal{A}_{i,j} = \frac{e^{(M_i N_j)}}{\sum_{r=1}^{n} e^{(M_r N_j)}}$. This $\mathcal{A}_{i,j}$ measures the input of the ith and j^{th} position. Similarly, the TSA attention is calculated as,

$$\mathcal{F}_{TSA}(K, Q, V) = soft\left(\frac{QK^T}{(d_k)^{1/2}}\right) V \tag{2}$$

where K, Q, V are just the features of $\mathcal{F}^t_{base}$ added with positional encoding and d_k is the dimensionality of any key or Query or value sequence (i.e., $d_k = |V| or |Q| or |K|$ and $soft(.)$ is the softmax activation function [13].) These attentions are operated at the latent space or base, and now, in final step, all these features are amalgamated at the latent space as,

$$\mathcal{F}_{SAA} = \psi_1 \mathcal{F}_{TSA} + \psi_2 \mathcal{F}_{GSA} + \mathcal{F}_{base} \tag{3}$$

where ψ_1 and ψ_2 are the scale parameters, respectively, and they control the importance assigned to each attention mechanism. Initially, they are assigned with null weights and gradually incremented to obtain a systematic consistency.

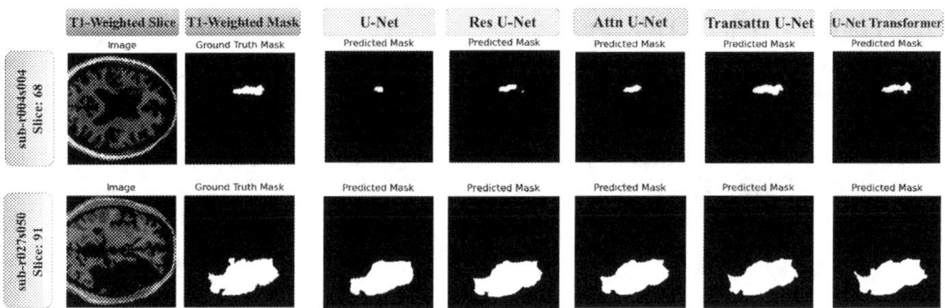

Fig. 2. 2D visualizations of the benchmarks between ground truth and predicted lesions for two subjects. As can be seen, we have two different sizes of stroke lesion subjects included for visualization (Subject ID: $sub-r027s050$ slice 91 and $sub-r004s004$ slice 68) of which one is small and the other being large. We display the predicted outputs of convolution and transformer-based 2D U-Net models for these subjects. All 2D models performed equally better but the U-Net transformer gave the finest boundaries as visible for both the subjects.

Table 5. The below table illustrates the performance of variants of 3D U-Net architectures. The models that are implied below are pure convolution-based architectures and the evaluation criteria implied are the same as Table 3; We report the performance of the model for the test set.

Method	Performance Metrics (3D Data)			
	Dice Score	IoU Score	Precision	Recall
U-Net [31]	0.450	0.350	0.584	0.444
Residual U-Net [42]	**0.504**	**0.393**	**0.585**	0.533
Attention U-Net [26]	0.469	0.369	0.498	**0.578**

U-Net Transformer: This method originated from the work by Petit *et al.* [28]. The authors impart self-attention and channel attention modules in this work to produce interpretative segmentation throughput. Fundamentally, the self-attention module uses Multi-head Self-Attention (MHSA) which is similar to Vaswani *et al.* [34], and this aims to acquire long-range structural information from the images that were downsampled to the latent-space. The underlying operation is quite similar to Eq. (2).

In the channel-attention module, the representations from skip connections (at each pooling step) are first applied with MHSA and then concatenate the features coming from latent space after each upsampling step. Thus this module is referred to as Multi-Head Channel-Attention (MHCA) as initially the input is transferred to MHSA and then concatenated with a cross-attention mechanism. The diagrammatic explanations are elucidated in Fig. 1.

4 Results and Discussion

In this section, we experiment with the aforementioned methods as summarized in Sect. 3. First, we evaluate the performance of 2D and 3D models. Later, we conducted the Wilcoxon test using the ground truth and predicted lesion volume for 3D U-Net models.

4.1 Results for 2D

Among the 2D U-Net convolution-based models the attention U-Net has proven to have a significant Dice score of 0.487 (with an extra verge of 7.0% dice score from baseline[3]). Whereas the hybrid transformer- and convolution-based models tend to provide a noteworthy performance of 0.583 and 0.572 dice scores. These models superseded 2D standard U-Net with an additional 15.5 and 16.6% of dice score respectively. All these results are illustrated in Table 4.

As there were no additional augmentations applied we can directly infer that adding self-attention components (latent space) such as TSA, MHSA, and GSA played a crucial role in providing significant performance with their cascaded attention [38].

In this regard, we have considered two subjects for visualizing the performance of each model in predicting lesions. In Fig. 2 we have displayed the potential of each model to segment small lesions (first row) and large lesions (second row). All the models were near good in segmenting the large volume of lesions but the U-Net Transformer is able to accurately delineate the boundaries of tissues from T1-weighted MRI. But, most of the models struggle to extract the small lesions. Hybrid models such as transformer-based architecture did perform well (comparatively) to a certain extent but, still, there is a wide scope for developing novel models.

4.2 Results for 3D

Now, we consider 3D U-Net style architectures which include standard U-Net, Residual, and Attention U-Net. Due to the added temporal relationship among the features in 3D convolution, the standard 3D U-Net was able to achieve a 0.45 dice score. Previously, in 2D modality, the convolution-based model did not achieve more than a 0.47 dice score. However, 3D modalities, both standard and residual U-Net have a decent increment in performance without any data augmentation [35]. The shift of modality from 2D to 3D, for Residual U-Net and standard U-Net, had an increment of 7.7% and 4.3% of dice score respectively. But, attention U-Net did not succeed in incriminating its performance by shifting from 2D to 3D. The reason behind it might be due to a lack of augmentations and an insufficient number of samples for training[4]. The results for these models under different performance metrics are illustrated in Table 5.

[3] In this paper we consider, standard U-Net to be our baseline for both 2D and 3D models respectively.

[4] The authors have experimented with various optimizers, learning schedulers, and many more hyperparameters.

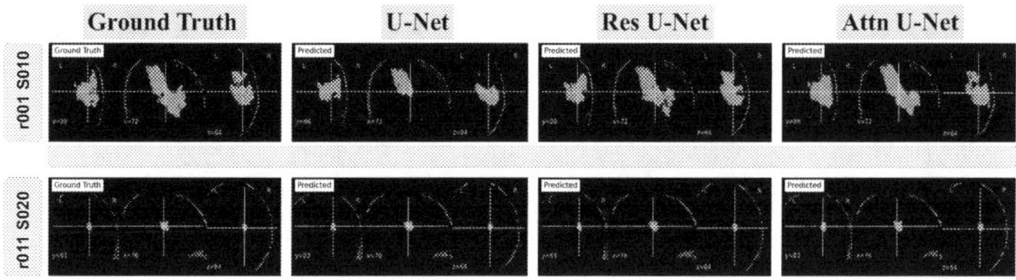

Fig. 3. The above visualization was considered from the test set (ID: $sub - r001s010$ and $sub - r011s020$) and compares three 3D U-Net models (standard, Residual, and Attention). For each model, the left part remains as ground truth and the right part is the model's predictions. In each image, the visualization elucidates the precise location of stroke in the brain using three axes (sagittal, coronal, and axial).

To specifically study the behaviour of 3D segmentation models we visualized certain test samples one of which is visualized in Fig. 3. We have considered two test samples and visualized each plot in three different axes. In each image, the first image describes the Coronal plane and the middle one is the Sagittal plane. Finally, the terminal one is an axial plane. The combination of these three views gives us an estimate of the 3-dimensional pattern of stroke lesions in the brain. As can be seen from Fig. 3, U-Net is unable to provide good segmentation outcomes. Though Residual and Attention U-Net were able to segment well but not on par with the mask.

Wilcoxon Signed Rank Test: Now, we also study the prominence of lesion volume using the ground truths [35]. This is achieved by conducting a statistical test, specifically, the Wilcoxon Signed Rank test, and studying whether the lesion volume distribution patterns for each test subject are similar or not[5]. Thus, we establish the results for all three 3D U-Nets (Refer Fig. 4). For U-Net and Residual U-Net, the test rejects the null hypothesis and whereas, for attention U-Net it accepts the test with a p-value of 0.54. The detailed results of the Wilcoxon test are detailed in the supplementary material. Also, we visualize box plots to assess the original and predicted volume distribution for the test samples as in Fig. 4.

The distribution of pixels changes after resizing them to a certain shape in the case of 2D. As 2D models are often shrunk and stretched, based on the model, and doing so can misguide the volume calculation. Thus, we cannot estimate the true volumes in such cases and that is the reason we have only reported for 3D models.

[5] This test could be understood as a non-parametric t-test. A detailed premier is provided in the supplementary material.

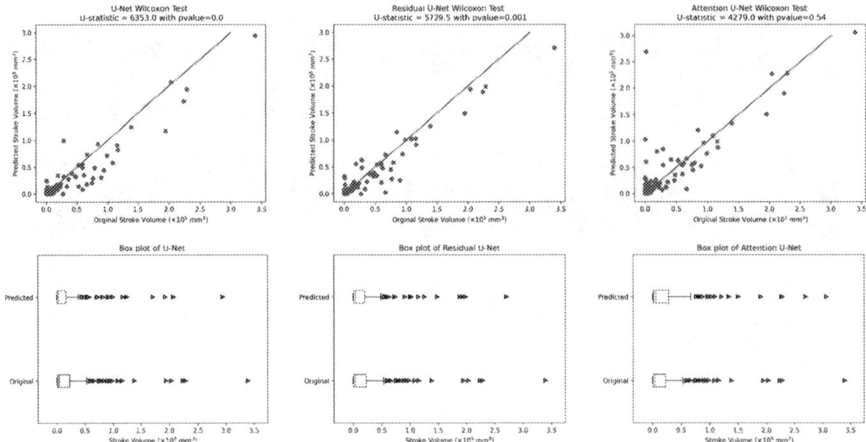

Fig. 4. The Wilcoxon test is carried out for all three 3D U-Net style architectures. The first row indicates a scatter plot and the second one indicates box plots of the predicted and actual stroke volume of the 3D models respectively. Specifically for the scatter plot. The ideal scenario must be the gray dots aligned with the red line. (Color figure online)

5 Limitations and Future Directions

In the analysis, we have considered a set of state-of-the-art models. But, there are certain limitations in the current work as described below:

- Our motto was to provide standard U-Net style models that are trained on ATLAS v2.0 without any augmentations. Thus, in this current work, we have not used any frameworks such as Deep Medic [20], nnU-Net [17], and MONAI [9].
- The current analysis is only done using models that have masks and so we achieved the results with supervision. Later, this work can be extended with weak-supervision [8,37] or self-supervision [16] approaches which can aid the learning of models in the absence of masks.
- This work does not focus on uncertainty or ambiguity in decision-making using generative models [6] [22] [30].
- Also, we did not address the issue of very small and disconnected lesions [16].

The limitations described above can be seen as future directions and they could contribute to the progressing field of Neuroimaging for Stroke prediction.

6 Conclusion

This paper fundamentally benchmarks variants of U-Net models on the ATLAS v2.0 dataset and deploys standard stroke lesion segmentation models which could be reproducible both for 2D and 3D brain images. We infer that current 2D or

3D brain imaging prediction requires much more attention towards developing hybrid models with the aid of *self-attention* mechanisms to improve the performance of the models. In the future, we tend to develop fine-grained segmentation models with data augmentation, multi-modality (Diffusion Weighted Imaging and T2-FLAIR), and cascaded attention mechanisms. We hope this research could progress and contribute to Stroke prediction.

Acknowledgement. The authors would like to acknowledge Manasa Kondamadugu for her invaluable coordination efforts throughout the project. Additionally, we extend our gratitude to IHub-Data, International Institute of Information and Technology, Hyderabad for their generous funding and support.

References

1. Achanta, R., Shaji, A., Smith, K., Lucchi, A., Fua, P., Süsstrunk, S.: Slic superpixels compared to state-of-the-art superpixel methods. IEEE Trans. Pattern Anal. Mach. Intell. **34**(11), 2274–2282 (2012)
2. Akkus, Z., Galimzianova, A., Hoogi, A., Rubin, D.L., Erickson, B.J.: Deep learning for brain mri segmentation: state of the art and future directions. J. Digit. Imaging **30**, 449–459 (2017)
3. Alom, M.Z., Yakopcic, C., Hasan, M., Taha, T.M., Asari, V.K.: Recurrent residual u-net for medical image segmentation. J. Med. Imaging **6**(1), 014006–014006 (2019)
4. Bahdanau, Dzmitry, K.C., Bengio, Y.: Neural machine translation by jointly learning to align and translate. In: ICLR (2014)
5. Baird, A.E., Warach, S.: Magnetic resonance imaging of acute stroke. J. Cerebral Blood Flow Metab. **18**(6), 583–609 (1998)
6. Baumgartner, C.F., et al.: PHiSeg: capturing uncertainty in medical image segmentation. In: Shen, D., et al. (eds.) MICCAI 2019. LNCS, vol. 11765, pp. 119–127. Springer, Cham (2019). https://doi.org/10.1007/978-3-030-32245-8_14
7. Bhalerao, M., Thakur, S.: Brain tumor segmentation based on 3D residual u-net. In: Crimi, A., Bakas, S. (eds.) BrainLes 2019. LNCS, vol. 11993, pp. 218–225. Springer, Cham (2020). https://doi.org/10.1007/978-3-030-46643-5_21
8. Cao, C., Liu, Z., Liu, G., Jin, S., Xia, S.: Ability of weakly supervised learning to detect acute ischemic stroke and hemorrhagic infarction lesions with diffusion-weighted imaging. Quant. Imaging Med. Surg. **12**(1), 321 (2022)
9. Cardoso, M.J., et al.: Monai: an open-source framework for deep learning in healthcare. arXiv preprint arXiv:2211.02701 (2022)
10. Chen, B., Liu, Y., Zhang, Z., Lu, G., Kong, A.W.K.: Transattunet: multi-level attention-guided u-net with transformer for medical image segmentation. arXiv preprint arXiv:2107.05274 (2021)
11. Çiçek, Ö., Abdulkadir, A., Lienkamp, S.S., Brox, T., Ronneberger, O.: 3D U-Net: learning dense volumetric segmentation from sparse annotation. In: Ourselin, S., Joskowicz, L., Sabuncu, M.R., Unal, G., Wells, W. (eds.) MICCAI 2016. LNCS, vol. 9901, pp. 424–432. Springer, Cham (2016). https://doi.org/10.1007/978-3-319-46723-8_49
12. Ciresan, D., Giusti, A., Gambardella, L., Schmidhuber, J.: Deep neural networks segment neuronal membranes in electron microscopy images. Adv. Neural Inf. Process. Syst. **25** (2012)

13. Elfadel, I.M., Wyatt Jr, J.L.: The "softmax" nonlinearity: derivation using statistical mechanics and useful properties as a multiterminal analog circuit element. Adv. Neural Inf. Process. Syst. **6** (1993)
14. Grady, L.: Random walks for image segmentation. IEEE Trans. Pattern Anal. Mach. Intell. **28**(11), 1768–1783 (2006)
15. He, K., Zhang, X., Ren, S., Sun, J.: Deep residual learning for image recognition. In: 2016 IEEE Conference on Computer Vision and Pattern Recognition (CVPR), pp. 770–778 (2016). https://doi.org/10.1007/978-3-319-46723-8_4910.1109/CVPR.2016.90
16. Huo, J., et al.: Mapping: model average with post-processing for stroke lesion segmentation. arXiv preprint arXiv:2211.15486 (2022)
17. Isensee, F., Jaeger, P.F., Kohl, S.A., Petersen, J., Maier-Hein, K.H.: nnu-net: a self-configuring method for deep learning-based biomedical image segmentation. Nat. Methods **18**(2), 203–211 (2021)
18. Isensee, F., Maier-Hein, K.H.: An attempt at beating the 3d u-net. arXiv preprint arXiv:1908.02182 (2019)
19. Johnson, W., Onuma, O., Owolabi, M., Sachdev, S.: Stroke: a global response is needed. Bull. World Health Organ. **94**(9), 634 (2016)
20. Kamnitsas, K., et al.: Efficient multi-scale 3d cnn with fully connected crf for accurate brain lesion segmentation. Med. Image Anal. **36**, 61–78 (2017)
21. Kim, J., et al.: Global stroke statistics 2019. Int. J. Stroke **15**(8), 819–838 (2020)
22. Kohl, S., et al.: A probabilistic u-net for segmentation of ambiguous images. Adv. Neural Inf. Process. Syst. **31** (2018)
23. Liew, S.L., et al.: A large, open source dataset of stroke anatomical brain images and manual lesion segmentations. Sci. Data **5**(1), 1–11 (2018)
24. Liew, S.L., et al.: A large, curated, open-source stroke neuroimaging dataset to improve lesion segmentation algorithms. Sci. data **9**(1), 320 (2022)
25. Nodirov, J., Abdusalomov, A.B., Whangbo, T.K.: Attention 3d u-net with multiple skip connections for segmentation of brain tumor images. Sensors **22**(17), 6501 (2022)
26. Oktay, O., et al.: Attention u-net: learning where to look for the pancreas. arXiv preprint arXiv:1804.03999 (2018)
27. Paing, M.P., Tungjitkusolmun, S., Bui, T.H., Visitsattapongse, S., Pintavirooj, C.: Automated segmentation of infarct lesions in t1-weighted mri scans using variational mode decomposition and deep learning. Sensors **21**(6), 1952 (2021)
28. Petit, O., Thome, N., Rambour, C., Themyr, L., Collins, T., Soler, L.: U-net transformer: self and cross attention for medical image segmentation. In: Lian, C., Cao, X., Rekik, I., Xu, X., Yan, P. (eds.) MLMI 2021. LNCS, vol. 12966, pp. 267–276. Springer, Cham (2021). https://doi.org/10.1007/978-3-030-87589-3_28
29. Qi, K., et al.: X-Net: brain stroke lesion segmentation based on depthwise separable convolution and long-range dependencies. In: Shen, D., et al. (eds.) MICCAI 2019. LNCS, vol. 11766, pp. 247–255. Springer, Cham (2019). https://doi.org/10.1007/978-3-030-32248-9_28
30. Rahman, A., Valanarasu, J.M.J., Hacihaliloglu, I., Patel, V.M.: Ambiguous medical image segmentation using diffusion models. In: Proceedings of the IEEE/CVF Conference on Computer Vision and Pattern Recognition, pp. 11536–11546 (2023)
31. Ronneberger, O., Fischer, P., Brox, T.: U-net: convolutional networks for biomedical image segmentation. In: Navab, N., Hornegger, J., Wells, W.M., Frangi, A.F. (eds.) MICCAI 2015. LNCS, vol. 9351, pp. 234–241. Springer, Cham (2015). https://doi.org/10.1007/978-3-319-24574-4_28

32. Sheng, M., Xu, W., Yang, J., Chen, Z.: Cross-attention and deep supervision unet for lesion segmentation of chronic stroke. Front. Neurosci. **16**, 836412 (2022)
33. Tomita, N., Jiang, S., Maeder, M.E., Hassanpour, S.: Automatic post-stroke lesion segmentation on mr images using 3d residual convolutional neural network. NeuroImage: Clin. **27**, 102276 (2020)
34. Vaswani, A., et al.: Attention is all you need. Adv. Neural Inf. Process. Syst. **30** (2017)
35. Verma, K., Kumar, S., Paydarfar, D.: Automatic segmentation and quantitative assessment of stroke lesions on mr images. Diagnostics **12**(9), 2055 (2022)
36. Wang, X., Han, S., Chen, Y., Gao, D., Vasconcelos, N.: Volumetric attention for 3D medical image segmentation and detection. In: Shen, D., et al. (eds.) MICCAI 2019. LNCS, vol. 11769, pp. 175–184. Springer, Cham (2019). https://doi.org/10.1007/978-3-030-32226-7_20
37. Wu, K., et al.: Weakly supervised brain lesion segmentation via attentional representation learning. In: Shen, D., et al. (eds.) MICCAI 2019. LNCS, vol. 11766, pp. 211–219. Springer, Cham (2019). https://doi.org/10.1007/978-3-030-32248-9_24
38. Wu, Z., Zhang, X., Li, F., Wang, S., Huang, L., Li, J.: W-net: a boundary-enhanced segmentation network for stroke lesions. Expert Syst. Appl. 120637 (2023)
39. Yu, W., Fang, B., Liu, Y., Gao, M., Zheng, S., Wang, Y.: Liver vessels segmentation based on 3d residual u-net. In: 2019 IEEE International Conference on Image Processing (ICIP), pp. 250–254. IEEE (2019)
40. Yu, W., Huang, Z., Zhang, J., Shan, H.: San-net: learning generalization to unseen sites for stroke lesion segmentation with self-adaptive normalization. Comput. Biol. Med. **156**, 106717 (2023)
41. Zhang, Y., Wu, J., Liu, Y., Chen, Y., Wu, E.X., Tang, X.: Mi-unet: multi-inputs unet incorporating brain parcellation for stroke lesion segmentation from t1-weighted magnetic resonance images. IEEE J. Biomed. Health Inf. **25**(2), 526–535 (2020)
42. Zhang, Z., Liu, Q., Wang, Y.: Road extraction by deep residual u-net. IEEE Geosci. Remote Sens. Lett. **15**(5), 749–753 (2018)
43. Zhou, Y., Huang, W., Dong, P., Xia, Y., Wang, S.: D-unet: a dimension-fusion u shape network for chronic stroke lesion segmentation. IEEE/ACM Trans. Comput. Biol. Bioinf. **18**(3), 940–950 (2019)

Towards Radiomics-Based Automated Disease Progression Assessment for Glioblastoma Patients

Yannick Suter[1,2,5(✉)], Flurina Schuhmacher[1,5], Ekin Ermis[2,5], Urspeter Knecht[3,5], Philippe Schucht[4,5], Roland Wiest[4,5], and Mauricio Reyes[1,2,5]

[1] ARTORG Center for Biomedical Engineering Research, University of Bern, Bern, Switzerland
yannick.suter@unibe.ch
[2] Department of Radiation Oncology, Inselspital, Bern University Hospital and University of Bern,Bern, Switzerland
[3] Radiology Department, Emmental Hospital, Burgdorf, Switzerland
[4] Department of Neurosurgery, Inselspital, Bern University Hospital, Bern, Switzerland
[5] Support Center for Advanced Neuroimaging, Inselspital, Bern University Hospital, Bern, Switzerland

Abstract. Glioblastoma is a highly infiltrative brain tumor with fast progression and poor prognosis for patients. Due to the rapid growth, close treatment response monitoring is key. In this study, we benchmark different machine learning approaches for automated progression classification with various radiomic feature sets extracted from longitudinal magnetic resonance imaging and classifiers. Our experiments show differences in robustness and performance and offer insights into common failure modes. The best ROC-AUC was achieved with a random forest classifier without feature selection (0.748), and the best F1 score was at 0.792 for an XGBoost classifier where features of the current time point and the change from the reference time point were provided. Analyzing misclassifications shows different behavior for statistical machine learning classifiers and Residual Neural Networks.

Keywords: Disease progression prediction · radiomics · MRI · longitudinal

1 Introduction

Glioblastoma (GBM) is a highly infiltrative brain tumor where patients have a median overall survival time of only 16 months. It is treated with maximum safe resection followed by chemo- and radiotherapy [28]. The fast tumor growth and poor prognosis make early detection of disease progression crucial. The current guidelines for treatment response assessment are outlined in the response

U. Baid et al. (Eds.): BrainLes 2023/SWITCH 2023, LNCS 14668, pp. 36–47, 2024.
https://doi.org/10.1007/978-3-031-76160-7_4

assessment in neuro-oncology criteria (RANO) [6]. Based on T1-weighted pre- and post-contrast (T1, T1c), T2-weighted, and T2-Fluid-Attenuated Inversion Recovery (FLAIR) follow-up Magnetic Resonance Imaging (MRI), the disease status is evaluated approximately every three months. The quantitative component of RANO considers the change of contrast-enhancing lesions above a measurability threshold, measured by a bi-dimensional product of diameters. A qualitative assessment is used for the T2-/FLAIR progression. The appearance of new lesions is also considered. The complexity and time-consuming aspect of clinical assessments has called for the development of machine and deep learning methods. The publicly available Brain Tumor Segmentation challenge dataset with pre-operative MRI has, for example, fueled research on tumor segmentation and overall survival prediction [2,19]. However, the lack of robustness of end-to-end pipelines is still an issue attributed to dataset size limitations, varying image acquisition parameters, and the complexity of the task. Radiomics-based approaches have shown promising levels of robustness and interpretability in cancer imaging tasks [21,24] but at the potential cost of reduced levels of model performance. Hence, their combination has been leveraged as a reasonable trade-off between average performance and robustness [8].

Specifically, for GBM patients, previous works have mainly focused on overall survival prediction [10,11,23] and progression-free survival prediction from single-time point imaging information [20], or pseudo vs. true progression classification [12]. Another study tried to learn GBM progression biomarkers [26]. Closest to our work is the study of [15] that uses longitudinal imaging information but relies on a temporal analysis of perfusion MR sequences, which are not readily available across centers, and does not use the RANO guidelines to define progression.

Based on the advancements in automated tumor segmentation and promising results of radiomics-based analysis in other neuroradiological tasks, we aim to benchmark automated disease progression classification. Based on a publicly available longitudinal dataset, we test a variety of statistical machine learning algorithms and a tabular deep learning method.

2 Materials and Methods

2.1 Data

We rely on the LUMIERE dataset for this study since it is currently the only publicly available dataset with longitudinal RANO labels [25]. It contains MRI data of 91 patients treated at a single center. We used the radiomic features derived from all time points in the dataset with all four MR images available to have automated tumor segmentations through HD-GLIO-AUTO [9,13]. We selected the segmentations stemming from this tool since its training includes a vast multi-centric pre- and post-operative dataset. A previous study found that the contrast-enhancing volume trend agreement to the automated segmentation was at 81.1%, setting an approximate upper boundary for the expected accuracy since we rely on these automated segmentations [27].

The RANO criteria define disease progression based on the imaging data at the current time point and a reference time point (nadir or baseline). This reference time point is selected as the study with the lowest tumor load. To provide a classification model with a similar amount of information as a clinician would consider, we concatenate the radiomic features of all follow-up scans ("current" timepoint) with those of the respective reference time point (or the difference to the current time point, see below). We also include an experiment where only the difference between the features of the two time points is provided to the classifier.

Because complete data is needed from follow-up studies and the reference time points, our final dataset comprises data from 75 patients with 360 time points. To account for a progression vs. non-progression model, we pooled the RANO ratings of complete response, partial response, and stable disease into the non-progression group. This yielded 230 time points rated as progression and 130 as non-progression. Please note that the RANO protocol handles pseudo-progression by revising the initial rating with findings on a subsequent follow-up study.

For each patient, between one and 16 follow-up time points were available, with a mean of 4.9 per patient. The maximum time since the reference time point was 241 weeks; the minimum was one week.

2.2 Radiomic Features

For this feasibility study, we focus on features extracted with the `PyRadiomics`-Package, which includes first-order, shape-based, gray level co-occurrence matrix (GLCM), gray level run length matrix (GLRLM), gray level size zone matrix (GLSZM), neighboring gray-tone difference matrix (NGTDM), and gray level dependence matrix (GLDM) features. These features were extracted for all four MRI sequences and HD-GLIO output labels (contrast-enhancing tumor and T2/FLAIR abnormality). Since the shape features only depend on the segmentation and not the MRI sequences, this feature type was only extracted for one MRI sequence. This resulted in 772 features for each time point. A simple zero imputation was used in the case of missing values (which can be caused by the absence of a segmentation label (true negative or false negative).

For this study, we relied on the pre-extracted features provided with the dataset. These were originally extracted after z-score normalization of the MRI images, scaling by a factor of 100 and intensity shifting by 300. The histogram bin width was set to 5 [25].

A better performance may be expected by optimizing the feature extraction to the task.

2.3 Feature Sets

We tested different feature sets to benchmark the robustness and performance of classifiers:

1. All features from the current time point concatenated with the difference between the current and reference time point features (1544 features, "Curr &

Delta"). This informs the classifier about the current tumor/image properties and the changes since the reference time point. We expect the difference to be sensitive to, e.g., different acquisition parameters. We suspect that there is already a high information content in the features from the current time point since the baseline/nadir tumor load is typically very low; so a large tumor in the current time point will very often be a case of progression.
2. Only the difference between the current and reference time point features (772 features, "Delta"). As in the first feature set, but without the added information about the current image/tumor feature state.
3. Selecting 24 features with a mutual information feature selector (MIFS) from the current and reference time points (24 features, "MIFS - OVerall"). This last feature number was selected following the recommendation by [21], allowing one feature per ten samples in the training data. By letting the feature selection choose freely from the current and reference time points, we already encountered an imbalance of the selected features favoring the current time point (evaluation in the results section).
4. As in (3), but without feature selection (1544 features, "No selection"). This was to test how the classifiers perform where many more features than samples are available.
5. Providing only the volumes of the contrast-enhancement and the T2/FLAIR abnormality for both time points (4 features, "Volumes"). This is closest to the RANO guidelines, minus the consideration of newly occurring lesions, where we know from previous experiments that longitudinal lesion counts are inconsistent with the current automated segmentation methods [27].

No information about the timing of the follow-up scans was included as a feature. This will likely lead to misclassifications in situations where the image-based assessment indicates progression, but the RANO guidelines force the assessment to be stable disease since the difference to the reference time point was less than three months. Including time information, on the other hand, may have led to over-emphasizing this feature since most patients will have a progressive disease at some point.

2.4 Classifiers

We benchmarked a wide array of classifiers for this task. We tested Random Forest classifiers (RF) [3], XGBoost [4], AdaBoost [7], Support Vector classifiers (SVC) [5], Multilayer Perceptrons (MLP) [22], Logistic Regression, and Explainable Boosting Machines (EBM) [17]. Motivated by competitive results of ResNet-like networks on tabular deep learning benchmarks [8], we also include such a neural network. We tested parameter settings for each feature set and classifier combination, as described in the next section.

2.5 Model Optimization and Evaluation

Due to the relatively low sample size, all methods are tested through three-fold grouped cross-validation and based on ten fixed seed values to evaluate stochasticity effects. The grouping was based on the patient, ensuring that data from the same patient was not used both during training and testing. Each split had roughly the same percentage of progression and non-progression classes. Each feature was z-score normalized to have zero mean and unit variance within each training split. For the experiment with feature selection, the selection was performed based on the training set of each split individually. Parameters were only tuned on the first fold to ensure a fair comparison and avoid data leakage. We ran 100 trials with `Optuna` [1] based on three-fold cross-validation on the first fold to find a suitable parameter setting for each classifier. The best parameter setting was chosen based on the highest ROC-AUC value. We explored the parameter settings in the following search space: RF and XGBoost: maximum tree depth from 2 to 32, number of classifiers from 50 to 550, step size of 20; AdaBoost: learning rate from 0.2 to 2, number of estimators as for RF; SVC and logistic regression: parameter C from 0.3 to 3; MLP: hidden layer size from 80 to 1000; EBMs: between 1 and 20 interactions, and a learning rate from 10^{-4} to 0.05. Since EBMs offer the possibility to enforce interactions, we added an experiment where we consider interactions between features from the current and reference time points and excluded features without interactions (referred to as "EBM - Interactions" in the results). The ResNet neural network tested consisted of two residual blocks with a main layer size of 128 and hidden layers with 256 elements. Dropout for the residual blocks and final classification layer was set at 0.2. The network was trained with binary cross-entropy loss, batch size 200, and learning rate set at 10^{-6} with the Adam optimizer [14]. Early stopping was implemented based on the loss on a 10% validation set from each split with a patience of 400 epochs for a maximum of 10000 epochs.

The code used for this study is available at https://github.com/ysuter/towardsgbmprogression.

3 Results and Discussion

3.1 Performance Evaluation

The results of our experiments are summarized in Fig. 1 and Table 1, with aggregations across all folds and seeds. The best mean AUC was achieved with an RF classifier without feature selection at 0.748 ± 0.053. The ResNet with the features from the current and difference to the reference time point features achieved the best balanced accuracy (0.678 ± 0.074). The best F1 score was observed with an XGBoost classifier, again using the current and difference feature set ("Curr & Delta"). The classifiers not using any feature selection were surprisingly competitive, considering the low sample size and the large number of features.

3.2 Feature Importances

We postulate that a classifier should, in theory, draw features from both the current and reference time point, considering how the ground truth was created relying on the RANO criteria. We analyzed the feature's importances with

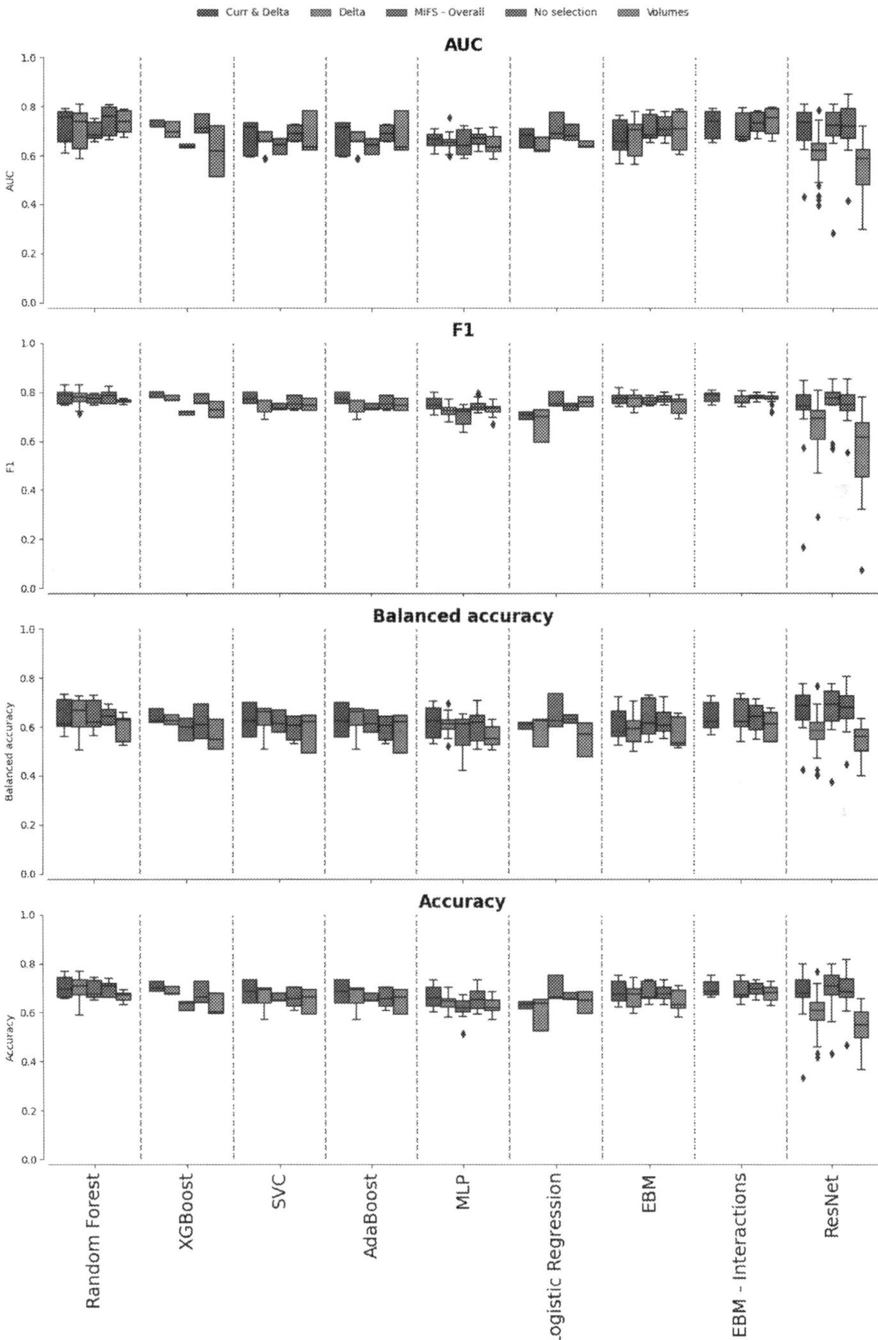

Fig. 1. Performance overview for AUC, F1, balanced accuracy, and accuracy for different classifiers and feature sets.

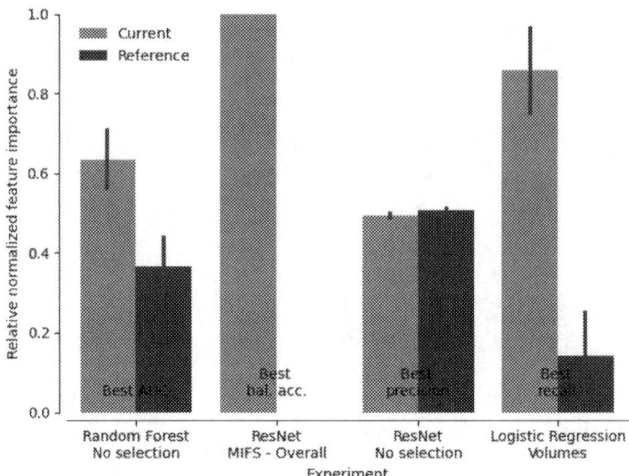

Fig. 2. Feature importances for the best-performing methods for AUC, balanced accuracy, precision, and recall. The bars show the normalized relative feature importance of all features of the current and reference time points. Bar height: mean, black error bars: standard deviation across folds and seeds.

permutation testing. Figure 2 shows the aggregated feature importances for the current and reference feature matrix parts across all folds and seeds for the best-performing methods for AUC, balanced accuracy, precision, and recall. The most balanced importance was observed for the ResNet without feature selection and the least for the classifiers after MIFS feature selection. Here, the MIFS selector already predominantly selected features from the current time point (97.2%). Many classifiers were able to reach competitive performance while disregarding the reference time point, potentially due to the fact that if a tumor volume of a certain size was present, progression is highly likely.

The contrast-enhancement volume was relatively unimportant compared to intensity-based features for the tested classifiers, most likely due to the large number of highly correlated features. Furthermore, we note that many higher-order features were correlated to the segmentation volume.

3.3 Misclassifications

Figure 3 shows the frequency of misclassifications for all methods and samples. Large dark stripes indicate especially hard samples where most classifiers failed to detect progression accurately. The ResNet classifiers seem to offer a different behavior from the statistical machine learning classifiers.

We went back to the neuroradiologist's rating to analyze the data from patients/time points where most classifiers were wrong. We found that 1) many times, the spacing to the reference time point was less than three months, forcing the rating to be stable disease even if signs of progression were observed, and 2) that progression occurred within the irradiated area. With the current proposals

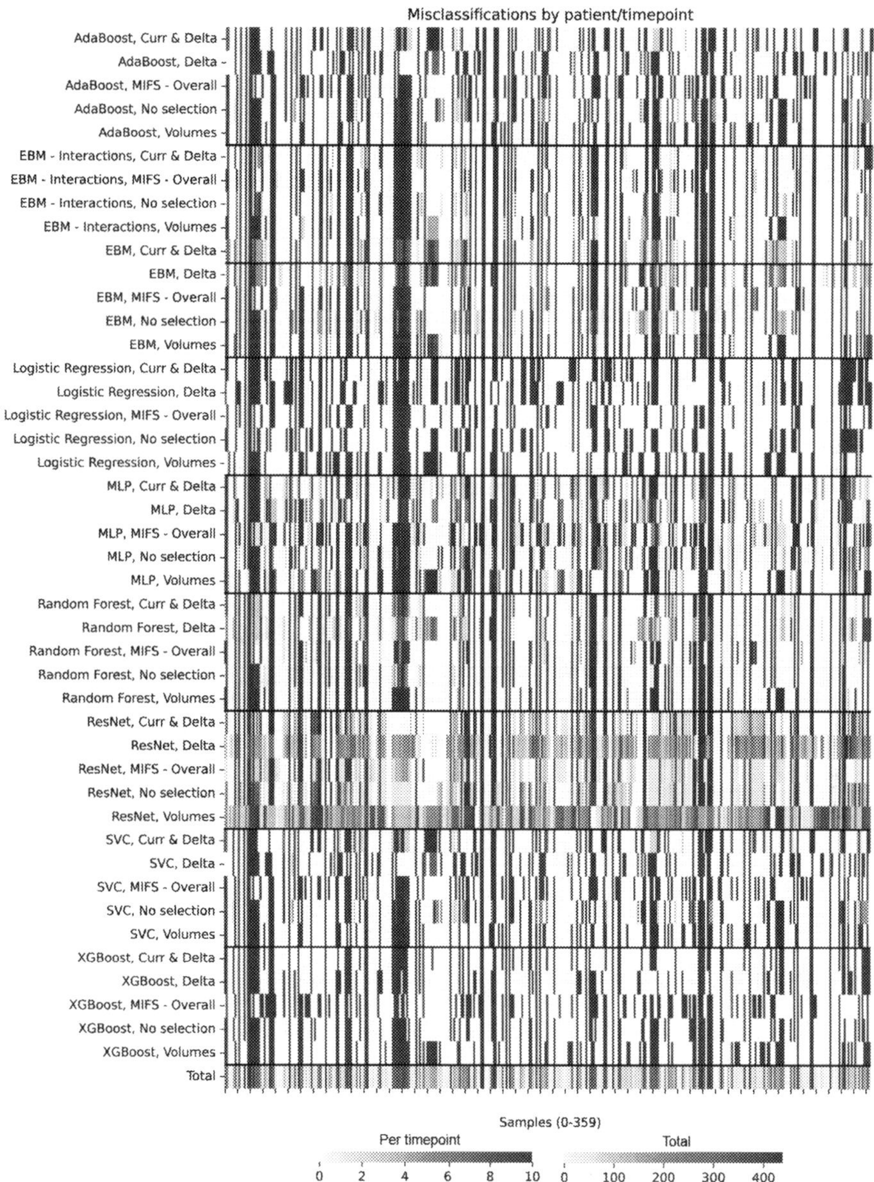

Fig. 3. The number of misclassifications for all tested methods across all patients and time points. Darker values represent more frequent misclassifications for a given sample. Please note that the visualized numbers are the sum across all folds for each time point and experiment. Black horizontal lines separate the different classifiers.

Table 1. Comparison of the progression classification performance for different feature sets and classifiers. The metrics are reported as the mean ± standard deviation across the three folds and ten seeds. The best mean overall performance is highlighted in green, and the best performance per classifier is marked in bold. If the performance of multiple feature sets were on par, the one with the lower standard deviation is marked.

Method	Feature set	AUC	Bal. acc.	F1
AdaBoost	Curr & Delta	0.678 ± 0.062	0.623 ± 0.062	**0.773 ± 0.021**
	Delta	0.656 ± 0.041	**0.626 ± 0.065**	0.744 ± 0.032
	MIFS - Overall	0.637 ± 0.027	0.62 ± 0.038	0.738 ± 0.011
	No selection	**0.696 ± 0.029**	0.601 ± 0.043	0.756 ± 0.024
	Volumes	0.678 ± 0.074	0.587 ± 0.069	0.749 ± 0.019
EBM	Curr & Delta	0.675 ± 0.065	0.611 ± 0.066	**0.774 ± 0.023**
	Delta	0.678 ± 0.069	0.591 ± 0.061	0.768 ± 0.026
	MIFS - Overall	0.708 ± 0.047	**0.632 ± 0.068**	0.765 ± 0.015
	No selection	**0.714 ± 0.041**	0.621 ± 0.052	0.771 ± 0.014
	Volumes	0.702 ± 0.067	0.57 ± 0.057	0.748 ± 0.033
EBM - forced interactions	Curr & Delta	0.728 ± 0.052	**0.641 ± 0.052**	0.781 ± 0.019
	MIFS - Overall	0.707 ± 0.053	0.64 ± 0.063	0.769 ± 0.019
	No selection	0.735 ± 0.036	0.638 ± 0.051	**0.781 ± 0.01**
	Volumes	**0.742 ± 0.049**	0.604 ± 0.055	0.774 ± 0.015
Logistic Regression	Curr & Delta	0.674 ± 0.032	0.607 ± 0.012	0.705 ± 0.012
	Delta	0.636 ± 0.027	0.591 ± 0.053	0.674 ± 0.058
	MIFS - Overall	**0.711 ± 0.047**	**0.654 ± 0.06**	**0.766 ± 0.027**
	No selection	0.69 ± 0.028	0.631 ± 0.014	0.739 ± 0.012
	Volumes	0.644 ± 0.012	0.554 ± 0.059	0.76 ± 0.015
Multilayer Perceptron	Curr & Delta	0.661 ± 0.031	**0.618 ± 0.06**	**0.752 ± 0.026**
	Delta	0.654 ± 0.03	0.61 ± 0.034	0.725 ± 0.023
	MIFS - Overall	0.65 ± 0.048	0.583 ± 0.061	0.706 ± 0.034
	No selection	**0.668 ± 0.025**	0.606 ± 0.061	0.743 ± 0.022
	Volumes	0.642 ± 0.038	0.561 ± 0.04	0.731 ± 0.02
Random Forest	Curr & Delta	0.729 ± 0.061	**0.649 ± 0.054**	0.783 ± 0.027
	Delta	0.713 ± 0.076	0.647 ± 0.067	0.778 ± 0.028
	MIFS - Overall	0.696 ± 0.033	0.642 ± 0.056	0.773 ± 0.017
	No selection	**0.748 ± 0.053**	0.643 ± 0.033	**0.784 ± 0.024**
	Volumes	0.735 ± 0.041	0.601 ± 0.05	0.763 ± 0.007
ResNet	Curr & Delta	0.719 ± 0.081	**0.678 ± 0.074**	0.736 ± 0.12
	Delta	0.607 ± 0.091	0.578 ± 0.08	0.66 ± 0.107
	MIFS - Overall	0.718 ± 0.097	0.678 ± 0.083	**0.77 ± 0.061**
	No selection	**0.724 ± 0.086**	0.676 ± 0.074	0.75 ± 0.058
	Volumes	0.546 ± 0.107	0.539 ± 0.066	0.562 ± 0.162
Support Vector Classifier	Curr & Delta	0.678 ± 0.062	0.623 ± 0.062	**0.773 ± 0.021**
	Delta	0.656 ± 0.041	**0.626 ± 0.065**	0.744 ± 0.032
	MIFS - Overall	0.637 ± 0.027	0.62 ± 0.038	0.738 ± 0.011
	No selection	**0.696 ± 0.029**	0.601 ± 0.043	0.756 ± 0.024
	Volumes	0.678 ± 0.074	0.587 ± 0.069	0.749 ± 0.019
XGBoost	Curr & Delta	**0.726 ± 0.013**	**0.639 ± 0.025**	**0.792 ± 0.01**
	Delta	0.703 ± 0.027	0.627 ± 0.017	0.774 ± 0.011
	MIFS - Overall	0.639 ± 0.007	0.592 ± 0.039	0.716 ± 0.006
	No selection	0.726 ± 0.034	0.619 ± 0.06	0.768 ± 0.018
	Volumes	0.619 ± 0.086	0.562 ± 0.051	0.728 ± 0.027

to update RANO to focus on post-treatment reference points, classification from image features may become easier with fewer treatment effects [16,29].

4 Conclusion

We benchmarked 44 feature sets and classifier combinations for automated GBM progression assessment using radiomic features. Even the best-performing models are far from providing accurate results for clinical routine use.

Further research should be directed at a detailed feature importance analysis and comparison with the RANO criteria. An extension to all four disease state classes would be interesting, although unfeasible with the currently available sample size, e.g., for a complete response to treatment. Using this method in a multi-center setting could give more information on a robustness benefit.

5 Outlook

As immediate follow-up experiments, we propose to test more elaborate feature normalization schemes considering the MRI parameters (e.g., ComBat, like in [18]) and try to leverage the ensembling of different approaches to minimize misclassifications.

Further experiments with ResNet-like architectures are necessary since we only considered rather small networks consisting of two residual blocks for this study. Furthermore, optimization of the network size, such as the number of residual blocks and the residual block sizes proved tricky with sweeps similar to those performed for the other classifiers since for some splits, the un-trained networks were already considered as best by Optuna.

Acknowledgments. We gladly acknowledge the Swiss Cancer Research funding (grant KFS-3979-08-2016) and the NVIDIA Corporation for donating a Titan Xp GPU. Computations were partly performed on Ubelix, the HCP cluster at the University of Bern.

References

1. Akiba, T., Sano, S., Yanase, T., Ohta, T., Koyama, M.: Optuna: a next-generation hyperparameter optimization framework. In: Proceedings of the 25th ACM SIGKDD International Conference on Knowledge Discovery and Data Mining (2019)
2. Bakas, S., et al.: Identifying the best machine learning algorithms for brain tumor segmentation, progression assessment, and overall survival prediction in the brats challenge. arXiv preprint arXiv:1811.02629 (2018)
3. Breiman, L.: Random forests. Mach. Learn. **45**, 5–32 (2001)
4. Chen, T., et al.: Xgboost: extreme gradient boosting. R package version 0.4-2 **1**(4), 1–4 (2015)
5. Cortes, C., Vapnik, V.: Support-vector networks. Mach. Learn. **20**, 273–297 (1995)

6. Ellingson, B.M., Wen, P.Y., Cloughesy, T.F.: Modified criteria for radiographic response assessment in glioblastoma clinical trials. Neurotherapeutics **14**(2), 307–320 (2017)
7. Freund, Y., Schapire, R.E.: A desicion-theoretic generalization of on-line learning and an application to boosting. In: Vitányi, P. (ed.) EuroCOLT 1995. LNCS, vol. 904, pp. 23–37. Springer, Heidelberg (1995). https://doi.org/10.1007/3-540-59119-2_166
8. Gorishniy, Y., Rubachev, I., Khrulkov, V., Babenko, A.: Revisiting deep learning models for tabular data. Adv. Neural. Inf. Process. Syst. **34**, 18932–18943 (2021)
9. Isensee, F., Petersen, J., Kohl, S.A., Jäger, P.F., Maier-Hein, K.H.: nnu-net: breaking the spell on successful medical image segmentation, **1**(1–8), 2 (2019). arXiv preprint arXiv:1904.08128
10. Islam, M., Wijethilake, N., Ren, H.: Glioblastoma multiforme prognosis: MRI missing modality generation, segmentation and radiogenomic survival prediction. Comput. Med. Imaging Graph. **91**, 101906 (2021)
11. Ismail, M., et al.: Radiomic deformation and textural heterogeneity (r-depth) descriptor to characterize tumor field effect: application to survival prediction in glioblastoma. IEEE Trans. Med. Imaging **41**(7), 1764–1777 (2022)
12. Jang, B.S., et al.: Machine learning model to predict pseudoprogression versus progression in glioblastoma using mri: a multi-institutional study (krog 18–07). Cancers **12**(9), 2706 (2020)
13. Kickingereder, P.: Automated quantitative tumour response assessment of mri in neuro-oncology with artificial neural networks: a multicentre, retrospective study. Lancet Oncol. **20**(5), 728–740 (2019)
14. Kingma, D.P., Ba, J.: Adam: a method for stochastic optimization. arXiv preprint arXiv:1412.6980 (2014)
15. Larsson, C., et al.: Prediction of survival and progression in glioblastoma patients using temporal perfusion changes during radiochemotherapy. Magn. Reson. Imaging **68**, 106–112 (2020)
16. Leao, D., Craig, P., Godoy, L., Leite, C., Policeni, B.: Response assessment in neuro-oncology criteria for gliomas: practical approach using conventional and advanced techniques. Am. J. Neuroradiol. **41**(1), 10–20 (2020)
17. Lou, Y., Caruana, R., Gehrke, J.: Intelligible models for classification and regression. In: Proceedings of the 18th ACM SIGKDD International Conference on Knowledge Discovery and Data Mining, pp. 150–158 (2012)
18. Mahon, R., Ghita, M., Hugo, G.D., Weiss, E.: Combat harmonization for radiomic features in independent phantom and lung cancer patient computed tomography datasets. Phys. Med. Biol. **65**(1), 015010 (2020)
19. Menze, B.H., et al.: The multimodal brain tumor image segmentation benchmark (brats). IEEE Trans. Med. Imaging **34**(10), 1993–2024 (2014)
20. Pak, E., et al.: Prediction of prognosis in glioblastoma using radiomics features of dynamic contrast-enhanced MRI. Korean J. Radiol. **22**(9), 1514 (2021)
21. Papanikolaou, N., Matos, C., Koh, D.M.: How to develop a meaningful radiomic signature for clinical use in oncologic patients. Cancer Imaging **20**, 1–10 (2020)
22. Rosenblatt, F.: The perceptron: a probabilistic model for information storage and organization in the brain. Psychol. Rev. **65**(6), 386 (1958)
23. Suter, Y., et al.: Deep learning versus classical regression for brain tumor patient survival prediction. In: Crimi, A., Bakas, S., Kuijf, H., Keyvan, F., Reyes, M., van Walsum, T. (eds.) BrainLes 2018. LNCS, vol. 11384, pp. 429–440. Springer, Cham (2019). https://doi.org/10.1007/978-3-030-11726-9_38

24. Suter, Y., et al.: Radiomics for glioblastoma survival analysis in pre-operative MRI: exploring feature robustness, class boundaries, and machine learning techniques. Cancer Imaging **20**, 1–13 (2020)
25. Suter, Y., Knecht, U., Valenzuela, W., Notter, M., Hewer, E., Schucht, P., Wiest, R., Reyes, M.: The lumiere dataset: longitudinal glioblastoma mri with expert rano evaluation. Sci. Data **9**(1), 768 (2022)
26. Suter, Y., Knecht, U., Wiest, R., Hewer, E., Schucht, P., Reyes, M.: Towards MRI progression features for glioblastoma patients: from automated volumetry and classical radiomics to deep feature learning. In: Kia, S.M., et al. (eds.) MLCN/RNO-AI -2020. LNCS, vol. 12449, pp. 129–138. Springer, Cham (2020). https://doi.org/10.1007/978-3-030-66843-3_13
27. Suter, Y., et al.: Evaluating automated longitudinal tumor measurements for glioblastoma response assessment. Front. Radiol. **3**, 1211859 (2023)
28. Weller, M., Le Rhun, E., Preusser, M., Tonn, J.C., Roth, P.: How we treat glioblastoma. ESMO Open **4**, e000520 (2019)
29. Wen, P.Y., et al.: Rano 2.0: proposal for an update to the response assessment in neuro-oncology (rano) criteria for high-and low-grade gliomas in adults (2023)

Domain Unlearning Boosts Lesion Segmentation Performance on Seen and Unseen MR Scanner Data

Domen Preložnik(✉) and Žiga Špiclin

Faculty of Electrical Engineering, University of Ljubljana, Tržaška Cesta 24, 1000 Ljubljana, Slovenia
{domen.preloznik,ziga.spiclin}@fe.uni-lj.si

Abstract. Inter-scanner variability was highlighted in the 2020 MAGNIMS consensus guidelines as most-detrimental factor in image acquisition with high impact on the diagnostic and prognostic quality of the MR scans. This study aimed to evaluate and compare the contributions of domain unlearning on white matter lesion segmentation from the MR scans. We used the MSSEG 2016 challenge dataset of 53 MS patients, where MR images were acquired on 4 different scanners, one of which was absent in the training split. Our approach was the state-of-the-art Swin UNETR segmentation model that was adopted for domain unlearning to better handle inter-scanner bias. Performance of lesion segmentation was evaluated according to challenge protocol and compared to three best challenge results and the state-of-the-art results of recently proposed Dense Residual UNET method. The baseline Swin UNETR model achieved comparable results to the three challenge methods, while our domain unlearning model consistently improved in all metrics versus the baseline model and achieved the highest Dice score among all tested methods. The principal impact of unlearning was in reducing false positive annotations, whereas performance consistently improved on seen and unseen scanner data, indicating that scanner-specific intensity artifacts do not overlap with the information required for lesion segmentation.

Keywords: lesion segmentation · unlearning · inter-scanner variability

1 Introduction

1.1 Description of Purpose

Inter-scanner variability (ISV) of Magnetic Resonance (MR) brain imaging was highlighted in the 2020 MAGNIMS consensus [1] as a single, most-detrimental factor with high impact on the diagnostic and prognostic quality of the obtained MR scans. The presence of disturbing factors as a consequence of the individual MR scanner and acquisition protocol characteristics has already been identified in the scientific community [2], and is reflected in the captured MR images in the form different noise level and distribution, contrast variations and artefacts. In the application of detection and delineation of pathological lesions in the white matter, from which quantitative biomarkers

U. Baid et al. (Eds.): BrainLes 2023/SWITCH 2023, LNCS 14668, pp. 48–56, 2024.
https://doi.org/10.1007/978-3-031-76160-7_5

of neurodegenerative diseases can be determined, the aforementioned variabilities represent a prevailing problem and a major obstacle in the clinical application of automated deep learning-based methods. The problem associated to this variability, and its impact on biomarker quantification, is clearly demonstrated when evaluating control images of the same patient on several different scanners [2].

Automated methods and tools to delineate brain tissue and pathological lesions are established as research tools, but not as clinical tools, as thus far they proved unreliable in new contexts, for example on images from a previously unseen MR scanner, and their results are consequently not reproducible. The research aim of this proposal is to improve the delineation of pathological lesions in the white matter using MR inter-scanner variability suppression technique through unlearning of scanner identifying information.

Lately, there has been a continued investigation of cross-domain multiple sclerosis (MS) lesion segmentation methods to improve the models' ability to generalize. Specifically, these methods aim to reduce the differences between domains by instructing the model to produce scanner-invariant characteristics [3, 4] training with synthetic images that conform to the distribution of the target scanners [5], and harmonizing data across scanners [6]. A fundamental requirement for these methods is to simultaneously incorporate data from various scanners into the framework.

In this work we propose the use of domain unlearning as a method of inter-scanner variability suppression and verify its performance on white-matter lesion segmentation task, achieving state-of-the-art results on the public MICCAI 2016 multiple sclerosis (MSSEG2016) challenge dataset [7]. With [8] in mind, we investigated improvements with adapted training protocol, whilst keeping model unaware of target domains.

2 Materials and Methods

2.1 Dataset

Dataset used for training and evaluation was the MSSEG2016 challenge dataset [7], which contains 3D magnetic resonance images of 53 patients with multiple sclerosis (MS) that were obtained from four different clinical centers (Centers 1, 3, 7, and 8) using four MR scanners with different field strengths (1.5T and 3T). The dataset includes 3D FLAIR, 3D T1-weighted (T1-w), 3D T1-w with gadolinium (GADO), 2D DP, and 2D T2 sequences for each patient. The images were divided into two subsets, with 15 patients for training and 38 patients for testing. The MR images of center 3 were not included in the training set, and thus represent the *unseen* data that will serve to assess the model's generalization capability and robustness.

The MS lesions in the dataset were manually delineated by seven experts, and a consensus mask was computed from their outputs for each patient using LOP-STAPLE algorithm. The voxel size of each MR scan varied from $1 \times 0.5 \times 0.5$ to $1.25 \times 1.04 \times 1.0$ mm. The MSSEG2016 challenge organizers provided raw and preprocessed MR images for each patient, whereas we used the former and applied to each modality the non-local means denoising, N4 bias correction and affine registration to the MNI152 atlas space.

2.2 Network Architecture

As a base model we used the Swin UNETR [9], which combines the Swin Transformer and the UNET and can therefore effectively handle both high- and low-level image features, making it a powerful tool for MR image segmentation. An important aspect of the Swin UNETR is the reduced number of parameters required for training, which is encouraging when working with relatively small datasets, as is the case with the MSSEG2016 dataset. The "R" in the UNETR stands for "residual", which indicates the residual connections used throughout the UNET architecture, which helps to mitigate the vanishing gradient problem and stabilizes model training.

In order to unlearn scanner-induced bias we mimicked the approach outlined in [8, 10], whereas we utilized the base Swin UNETR bottleneck and the fully connected feature output, to train an auxiliary convolutional neural network (CNN) as the domain classifier. Its aim was to determine the MR scanner ID as given in the training dataset. Input to the auxiliary CNN classifier were the feature maps of the Swin UNETR bottleneck and its fully connected output, that first passed through a down sampling stream of convolutional, ReLu activation and max-pooling layers to match the input feature map dimensions; next, the size-matched feature maps were concatenated and then passed to a multiple perceptron type of a classifier, with 3 output classes corresponding to IDs of scanners of centers 1, 7 and 8. The network architecture for unlearning is displayed in Fig. 1.

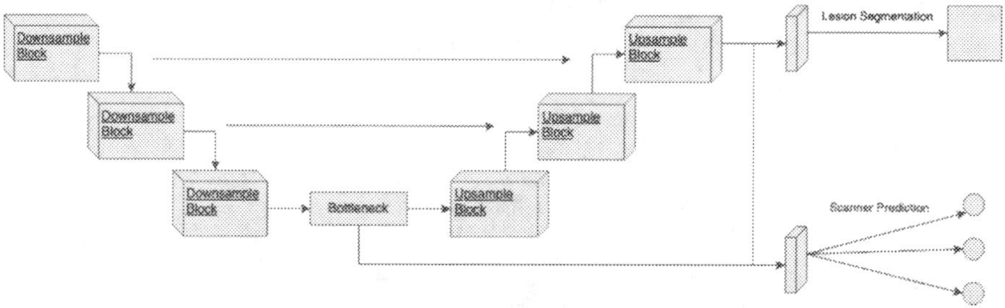

Fig. 1. The unlearning network architecture assembling the Swin UNETR for lesion segmentation and the auxiliary CNN for scanner (domain) classification.

2.3 Training Procedure

The Swin UNETR model entails the encoder, decoder, and predictor submodules. Training of the Swin UNETR was performed according to Algorithm 1 in two phases; in first, all submodules of the Swin UNETR model and the domain classifier were trained by minimizing the Dice loss and the categorical cross entropy loss, respectively. After a certain number of epochs, the first phase was extended with the confusion loss computed based on the domain classifier's output, followed by an update of the weights of the encoder and decoder submodules of the Swin UNETR based on confusion loss backpropagation, during which the domain classifier's weights were not updated.

Algorithm 1. Swin UNETR training procedure.

```
while epoch < max epochs:
  a: forward pass of input data through Swin UNETR model
  b: compute dice loss
  c: backpropagate Dice loss to Swin UNETR encoder, decoder and
     predictor
  d: forward pass the Swin UNETR output to domain classifier
  e: compute cross entropy loss
  f: backpropagation of cross entropy loss to domain classifier
  if epoch > epochs_start_unlearning:
    g: compute confusion loss
    h: backpropagate confusion loss to Swin UNETR encoder and decoder
  i: increment epoch
```

By minimizing the confusion loss, the domain classifier strived to achieve a uniform output class probability. In case of 3 target domains (i.e., 3 scanners IDs), the optimal domain classifier output would be 1/3 for each domain, thus minimizing the confusion loss. Contrary to the computation of the confusion loss in [10], we used categorical cross entropy with domain outputs as predictions and targets as a vector of equal distribution for all classes. The rationale behind having a target vector with an equal distribution for each class in domain adaptation is to maximize the confusion of the domain predictor about the source domain. This type of confusion loss computation enables model to be less prone to varying dataset domain distributions, whilst not always punishing model for correct source domain prediction, but rather to strive making models output uniform across all domain classes. This leads to the predictor outputting equal probabilities (1/N; N – number of source domains) for all classes. Class probabilities were thus as described:

$$P_i = \frac{1}{N}, \tag{1}$$

where i denotes the source domain class. The confusion loss was backpropagated through the Swin UNETR encoder and decoder parts, but not the predictor, as indicated in step h of Algorithm 1.

Training was carried out for both training phases until convergence was reached for the Swin UNETR model's Dice loss. Best results were obtained at epochs 183 and 2279 for the first and second phase, respectively. Figure 2 and Fig. 3 show the convergence curves of the classification accuracy and confusion loss values for the two phases (stage 1: figures in the Fig. 2, unlearning stage: figures in Fig. 3), where the y-axis represents the value of the measure that appears in the title of the plot and the x-axis shows the associated epoch number.

Clearly, the model unlearning process may adversely affect the primary segmentation task, therefore a carefully selected balance of the two associated loss functions was needed to obtain a satisfactory result. With trial and error, proper loss function weights were determined, in which the main goal of lesion segmentation was improved, for either source or target domain.

2.4 Evaluation and Metrics

Evaluation of the proposed method was performed according to the setup as used by the MSSEG2016 challenge organizers, using their proposed train and test dataset split. This

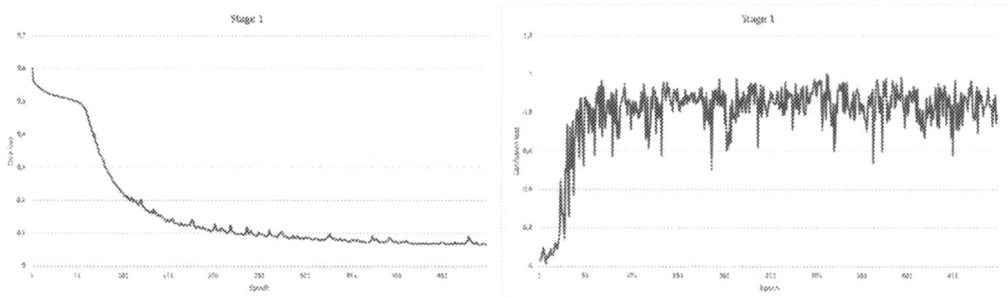

Fig. 2. Convergence curves of stage 1 (pre-unlearning stage) Dice and confusion losses respectively. X-axis represents the associated epoch number.

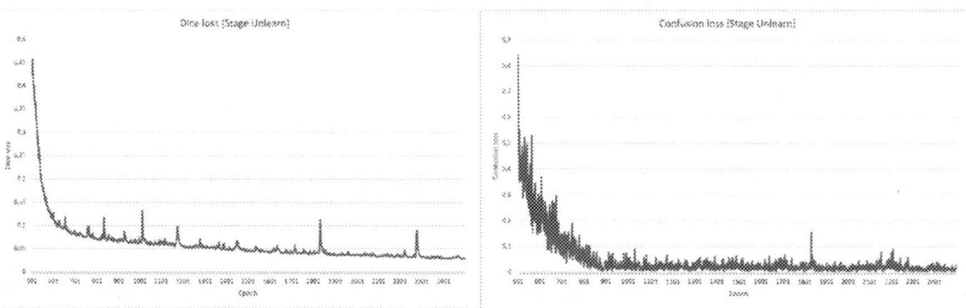

Fig. 3. Convergence curves of unlearning stage Dice and confusion losses respectively. X-axis represents the associated epoch number.

enables direct comparison to the state-of-the-art approaches using the same evaluation protocol, which involved the assessment of:

1. Dice similarity coefficient (DSC) computed between the predicted and consensus ground truth segmentation mask.
2. F1 score evaluating lesion detection and segmentation performance based on the number of correctly recognized lesions, regardless of the precision of their contours.
3. Positive predictive value (PPV) measuring the proportion of true positive predictions among all positive lesion voxels.
4. Sensitivity and specificity measured the overlap of lesion and non-lesion class.

We conducted an ablation study to calculate all beforementioned metrics. We evaluated the impact of each component of the system, as we ran these computations for the basic Swin UNETR model, as for versions of the model that had additional enhancements – a classifier and a confusion loss backpropagation.

Since our approach aims to perform domain information suppression through unlearning with the goal to improve generalization capacity on unseen new scanner data, we identified three best performing teams 6, 8 and 14 in the MSSEG2016 challenge results [7], according to the results achieved on the unseen scanner data from the test set (i.e. scanner data from Center 3). The recent and state-of-the-art Dense Residual UNET [11], and the basic and unlearnt Swin UNETR method were also comparatively evaluated.

3 Results

Teams 6, 8 and 14 achieved respective 0.568, 0.555 and 0.562 Dice score values on the unseen scanner (Center 3) data, whereas the average Dice score value across all challenge participants for the unseen scanner was substantially lower at 0.3794 [12]. Table 1 reports the evaluation results of the tested method and of Teams 6, 8, and 14 from the MSSEG2016 challenge.

The proposed method, i.e., the Swin UNETR Unlearn, achieved the highest overall Dice score of 0.678 among all tested methods. Compared to the other teams and models, the Swin UNETR Unlearn demonstrated improved performance by accurately identifying the TPs and, at the same time, reducing the number of FPs.

The original Swin UNETR achieved a Dice score of 0.638, lower than that of the Team 14 and of the Dense Residual U-net, while using unlearning, the score improved to 0.678. This indicates that the unlearning procedure substantially improved performance compared to the original Swin UNETR model, mainly through improving the PPV value (higher number of TPs and lower number of FPs).

Table 1. Results comparison between three MSSEG2016 challenge teams, Dense Residual UNET [11], Swin UNETR and our proposed Swin UNETR with domain unlearning.

	DSC	F1	PPV	Sensitivity	Specificity
Team 6	0.591*	0.386*	0.579*	0.660*	0.9997
Team 8	0.572*	0.451*	**0.699**	0.522*	**0.9998***
Team 14	0.639	0.504*	0.652	0.712	**0.9998***
Dense Residual U-Net	0.672	**0.588**	0.652	**0.744**	0.9997
Swin UNETR	0.638*	0.527	0.610*	0.742*	0.9994*
Swin UNETR Unlearn	**0.678**	0.563	**0.699**	0.710	0.9996

*Mean significantly different ($p < 0.05$) compared to Swin UNETR Unlearn approach according to Wilcoxon signed-rank test

Unlearning the base Swin UNETR model enhanced overall performance of lesion segmentation. Table 2 shows performance gain for each individual center, as well as the average across all centers. Looking at the metric values, we see that for each center, the DSC, F1 score, and PPV were improved from the original to the unlearning based version. The magnitude of the improvement varied across centers and across metrics. Looking at Center 3, which represent the scanner data not seen during model training, we can see that the Dice score value increased from 0.484 to 0.566, the F1 score increased from 0.292 to 0.405, and the PPV from 0.426 to 0.522.

Visual inspection of the segmentation results revealed that unlearning has successfully reduced noise and artifacts in medical image segmentation. The resulting segmentation maps show fewer segmentation artifacts and less spurious noisy pixels, indicating an overall improvement in the accuracy and robustness to scanner induced artifacts. One such example can be seen in Fig. 4.

Table 2. Evaluation of Dice, F1 and PPV score values for the base and unlearnt Swin UNETR model.

	Dice Score		F1 Score		PPV	
	Original	Unlearn	Original	Unlearn	Original	Unlearn
Center 1	0.722	**0.735**	0.599	**0.625**	0.721	**0.810**
Center 3	0.484	**0.566**	0.292	**0.405**	0.422	**0.522**
Center 7	0.656	**0.678**	**0.635**	0.618	0.622	**0.690**
Center 8	0.659	**0.707**	0.547	**0.577**	0.637	**0.740**
Average	0.638	**0.678**	0.527	**0.563**	0.610	**0.699**

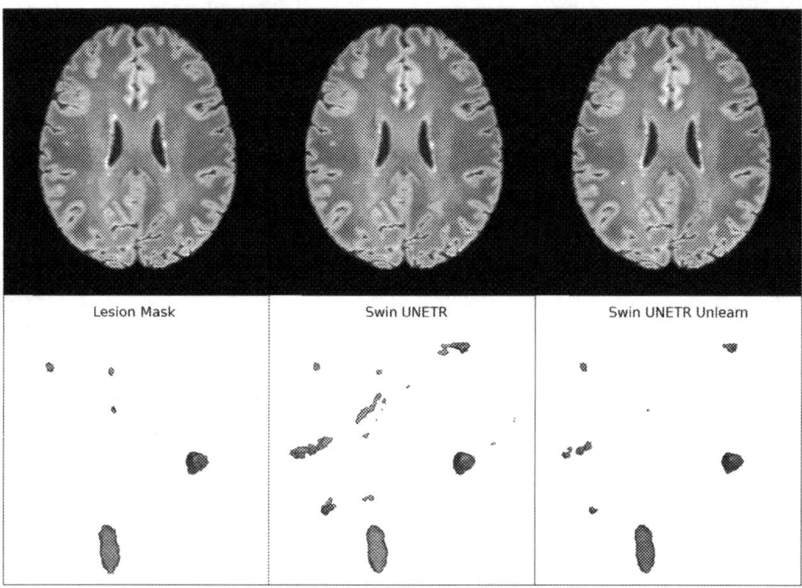

Fig. 4. Comparison of segmentation masks (*from left to right*): reference, original Swin UNETR, and Swin UNETR Unlearn. *Yellow arrows* indicate false positives due to scanner-induced periventricular hyperintensities. (Color figure online)

4 Discussion

Main contributions of this work are implementation and development of domain adaptation network using SOTA DL model, the Swin UNETR, and enhancing it with MR scanner bias unlearning loop; using cross entropy loss with 1/N per class distribution in domain classifier loss function; ablation study using externally validated tools provided in MSSEG2016 Challenge.

In regards to domain adaptation as previously pointed out in [10, 13], we have similarly achieved results out-performing base model (Swin UNETR in our case) utilizing confusion loss backpropagation. Unlike the methods described in the reference articles, our approach involved a distinct computation of the confusion loss, aiming to consistently predict similar probabilities across all output domains. Consequently, our method was not as heavily constrained by unequal representations of input domains as previous models.

Our results show that the Swin UNETR model with added MR scanner bias unlearning consistently outperformed the original Swin UNETR. Additionally, the Swin UNETR showed improved segmentation when using the test sub subset, with previously seen scanner data, potentially indicating that scanner-specific intensity information does not overlap with the information required for the lesion segmentation task. Whilst, we proved that unlearning with a limited set of source domains improved target domain score, a question arises, whether increasing the number of source domains would contribute to improved results of target domain lesion segmentation. With confusion loss being computed as proposed, class probabilities (as referenced in Eq. 1) would be represented accordingly, whilst discrepancy between per-domain inputs would become smaller, therefore performance may be impacted, due to lack of domain-specific characteristics.

We believe that with substantial improvement in lesion segmentation provided by the Swin UNETR Unlearn model, we demonstrated that unlearning scanner-specific variability represents a vitally important contribution to automated and versatile deep-learning-based lesion segmentation. In regard to MAGNIMS Consensus [1], we have improved model generalization that could potentially improve DL-based lesion segmentation to some extent, and thus make different-scanner acquisitions less impactful on actual medical diagnosis.

References

1. Sastre-Garriga, J., et al.: MAGNIMS consensus recommendations on the use of brain and spinal cord atrophy measures in clinical practice. Nat. Rev. Neurol. **16**(3), 3 (2020). https://doi.org/10.1038/s41582-020-0314-x
2. Akhondi-Asl, A., Hoyte, L., Lockhart, M.E., Warfield, S.K.: A logarithmic opinion pool based STAPLE algorithm for the fusion of segmentations with associated reliability weights. IEEE Trans. Med. Imaging **33**(10), 1997–2009 (2014). https://doi.org/10.1109/TMI.2014.2329603
3. Kamnitsas, K., et al.: Unsupervised domain adaptation in brain lesion segmentation with adversarial networks. arXiv (2016). https://doi.org/10.48550/arXiv.1612.08894
4. Ackaouy, A., Courty, N., Vallée, E., Commowick, O., Barillot, C., Galassi, F.: Unsupervised domain adaptation with optimal transport in multi-site segmentation of multiple sclerosis lesions from MRI data. Front. Comput. Neurosci. **14** (2020). Accessed 24 May 2022. https://doi.org/10.3389/fncom.2020.00019
5. Palladino, J.A., Slezak, D.F., Ferrante, E.: Unsupervised domain adaptation via CycleGAN for white matter hyperintensity segmentation in multicenter MR images. arXiv (2020). https://doi.org/10.48550/arXiv.2009.04985
6. Dewey, B.E., et al.: DeepHarmony: a deep learning approach to contrast harmonization across scanner changes. Magn. Reson. Imaging **64**, 160–170 (2019). https://doi.org/10.1016/j.mri.2019.05.041
7. Commowick, O., et al.: Multiple sclerosis lesions segmentation from multiple experts: the MICCAI 2016 challenge dataset. Neuroimage **244**, 118589 (2021). https://doi.org/10.1016/j.neuroimage.2021.118589

8. Sundaresan, V., Zamboni, G., Dinsdale, N.K., Rothwell, P.M., Griffanti, L., Jenkinson, M.: Comparison of domain adaptation techniques for white matter hyperintensity segmentation in brain MR images. Med. Image Anal. **74**, 102215 (2021). https://doi.org/10.1016/j.media.2021.102215
9. Hatamizadeh, A., Nath, V., Tang, Y., Yang, D., Roth, H., Xu, D.: Swin UNETR: swin transformers for semantic segmentation of brain tumors in MRI images. arXiv (2022). https://doi.org/10.48550/arXiv.2201.01266
10. Dinsdale, N.K., Jenkinson, M., Namburete, A.I.L.: Deep learning-based unlearning of dataset bias for MRI harmonisation and confound removal. Neuroimage **228**, 117689 (2021). https://doi.org/10.1016/j.neuroimage.2020.117689
11. Sarica, B., Seker, D.Z., Bayram, B.: A dense residual U-net for multiple sclerosis lesions segmentation from multi-sequence 3D MR images. Int. J. Med. Inf. **170**, 104965 (2023). https://doi.org/10.1016/j.ijmedinf.2022.104965
12. Commowick, O., et al.: Objective evaluation of multiple sclerosis lesion segmentation using a data management and processing infrastructure. Sci. Rep. **8**(1), 1 (2018). https://doi.org/10.1038/s41598-018-31911-7
13. Corral Acero, J., Sundaresan, V., Dinsdale, N., Grau, V., Jenkinson, M.: A 2-step deep learning method with domain adaptation for multi-centre, multi-vendor and multi-disease cardiac magnetic resonance segmentation. In: Puyol Anton, E., et al. (eds.) Statistical Atlases and Computational Models of the Heart. M&Ms and EMIDEC Challenges in LN CS, pp. 196–207. Springer, Cham (2021). https://doi.org/10.1007/978-3-030-68107-4_20

Primitive Simultaneous Optimization of Similarity Metrics for Image Registration

Diana Waldmannstetter[1,2(✉)], Benedikt Wiestler[3], Julian Schwarting[3], Ivan Ezhov[1,4], Marie Metz[3], Spyridon Bakas[5,6,7], Bhakti Baheti[5,6,7], Satrajit Chakrabarty[8], Daniel Rueckert[9,10], Jan S. Kirschke[3], Rolf A. Heckemann[11], Marie Piraud[12], Bjoern H. Menze[2], and Florian Kofler[1,3,4,12]

[1] Department of Informatics, Technical University of Munich, Munich, Germany
diana.waldmannstetter@tum.de

[2] Department of Quantitative Biomedicine, University of Zurich, Zurich, Switzerland

[3] Department of Diagnostic and Interventional Neuroradiology, School of Medicine, Klinikum rechts der Isar, Technical University of Munich, Munich, Germany

[4] TranslaTUM - Central Institute for Translational Cancer Research, Technical University of Munich, Munich, Germany

[5] Center for Artificial Intelligence and Data Science for Integrated Diagnostics (AI2D) and Center for Biomedical Image Computing and Analytics (CBICA), University of Pennsylvania, Philadelphia, PA, USA

[6] Department of Pathology and Laboratory Medicine, Perelman School of Medicine, University of Pennsylvania, Philadelphia, PA, USA

[7] Department of Radiology, Perelman School of Medicine, University of Pennsylvania, Philadelphia, PA, USA

[8] Department of Electrical and Systems Engineering, Washington University in St. Louis, St. Louis, MO, USA

[9] Artificial Intelligence in Healthcare and Medicine, Technical University of Munich, Munich, Germany

[10] Department of Computing, Imperial College London, London, UK

[11] Department of Medical Radiation Sciences, University of Gothenburg, Gothenburg, Sweden

[12] Helmholtz AI, Helmholtz Zentrum München, Munich, Germany

Abstract. Even though simultaneous optimization of similarity metrics is a standard procedure in the field of semantic segmentation, surprisingly, this is much less established for image registration. To help closing this gap in the literature, we investigate in a complex multi-modal 3D setting whether simultaneous optimization of registration metrics, here implemented by means of primitive summation, can benefit image registration. We evaluate two challenging datasets containing collections

B. H. Menze and F. Kofler—Equal contribution.

Supplementary Information The online version contains supplementary material available at https://doi.org/10.1007/978-3-031-76160-7_6.

U. Baid et al. (Eds.): BrainLes 2023/SWITCH 2023, LNCS 14668, pp. 57–68, 2024.
https://doi.org/10.1007/978-3-031-76160-7_6

of pre- to post-operative and pre- to intra-operative Magnetic Resonance (MR) images of glioma. Employing the proposed optimization, we demonstrate improved registration accuracy in terms of *Target Registration Error (TRE) o* on expert neuroradiologists' landmark annotations.

Keywords: Registration · Brain Tumor · Similarity Metric · Loss Function · Glioma

1 Introduction

The standard treatment for glioma is an *operative procedure (OP)* aiming to remove the tumor in full. Clinicians measure the success of surgery by comparing pre- and post-operative scans. Furthermore, this comparison is required for subsequent treatment planning, such as radiation therapy. Image registration techniques can enhance this process by providing a direct overlay of the differing structures. Enormous tissue shift and consequential missing correspondences mark a common side effect of tumor resection and pose a major challenge in registering pre- to post-operative images. The same holds true for intra-operative imaging in order to keep track of the surgery progress. A fast and accurate image registration method is beneficial for the precise estimation of tumor resection. Additionally, image registration is an important part of the preprocessing for segmentation algorithms [15,16]. Moreover, registration can be part of the segmentation algorithm itself [11]. Recent advances in the field of *Deep Learning (DL)* also benefited medical image registration. Methods like *VoxelMorph (VM)* [6], *LapIRN* [19], and *TransMorph* [9] have demonstrated that unsupervised deformable image registration is a promising alternative to frameworks based on iterative optimization algorithms like *Symmetric Normalization (SyN)* from *Advanced Normalization Tools (ANTs)* [3], *Free-Form Deformation (FFD)* [21] or toolboxes like Elastix [13]. *DL* methods provide comparable performance while significantly improving processing time. Within the scope of the *Brain Tumor Sequence Registration Challenge (BraTS-Reg)* [4], there has also been considerable development of registration algorithms for MR brain images before and after tumor resection [8,12,17,18,25]. Unsupervised *Deformable Registration Network (DRN)* can nicely register healthy brain scans [6,9,19]; however, they frequently struggle with large pathologies. Therefore, *Instance-Specific Optimization (IO) p* proved to be advantageous to mitigate major deformations [18,25]. Existing deep learning registration algorithms usually make use of a single similarity metric, often coupled with a smoothing regularization based on the deformation field, to be optimized in the loss function [6,19]. However, there is only limited literature investigating the combination of multiple similarity metrics to improve registration results [1,2,7,10,22,23,26].

In this work, we extend an unsupervised *DRN* using a combination of image similarity metrics, which are optimized simultaneously in the loss function. We benchmark the performance of our approach against the baseline on two challenging datasets of pre- to post-operative as well as pre- to intra-operative brain tumor images. Furthermore, we compare our approach to established reference methods, achieving competitive results. Following [6,18,25], we opt for instance-specific optimization in addition to the *DRN*. We demonstrate that the simultaneous optimization of two similarity metrics can improve registration accuracy in terms of *TRE* on expert landmark annotations.

2 Methods

Our workflow consists of three steps. First, we train a *Deformable Registration Network (DRN)*, followed by *Instance-Specific Optimization (IO)* at test time. Both *DRN* and *IO* optimize the same loss function. We then evaluate the registration performance in terms of *Target Registration Error (TRE)*.

2.1 Unsupervised Deformable Registration

We start our approach with a *DRN*, similar to [6]. Given two 3D images, a source image X and a target image Y, the network models the following function $f_\theta(X, Y) = u$, where the displacement field u, aligning X and Y, is defined bidirectionally, leading to $u_{x,y} = f_\theta(X, Y)$ and $u_{y,x} = f_\theta(Y, X)$ with θ being a set of learning parameters. X and Y are then warped with the respective displacement field using a spatial transform. While many *Convolutional Neural Network (CNN)*-based models are applicable here, like [6], we opt for a *U-Net*-like architecture with encoder, decoder and skip connections. The network architecture is based on an early implementation of *VM*, see GitHub implementation. The loss function comprises two main components, which are an image similarity metric and a smoothness regularizer for the displacement field. In addition to optimizing a single similarity metric as part of the loss function, we opt for optimizing multiple metrics simultaneously. An overview of the workflow is shown in Fig. 1.

2.2 Proposed Combined Loss Function

We define the objective function L for bidirectional training as follows:

$$L = \sum_{n=1}^{N} \left(L_{Sim_n}^{forward} \cdot \omega_n + L_{Sim_n}^{backward} \cdot \omega_n \right) + L_{Reg} \cdot \lambda \tag{1}$$

where N is the number of similarity metrics L_{Sim}, L_{Reg} is the regularization term, and the respective weights are denoted by ω_n and λ.

2.3 Instance-Specific Optimization

Since the registration results of a plain *DRN* might not always be sufficient, especially in the case of pathologies, *IO* is added in order to further refine the registration. Similar to [6], we take the output displacement field of *DRN* as initialization for a gradient-descent based iterative optimization on each test scan individually, following the initial training process. This technique optimizes the same loss function that is used for *DRN*. An overview of the complete method is given in Fig. 1.

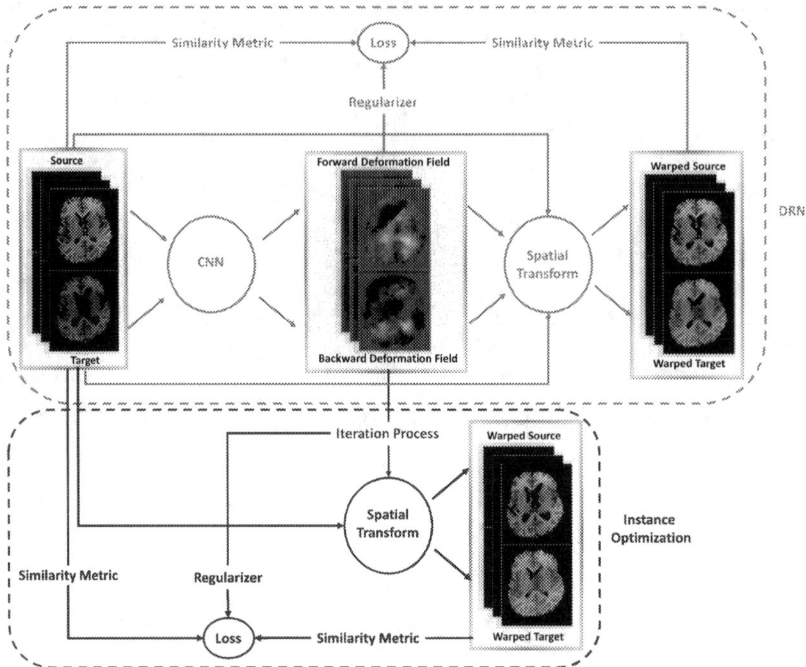

Fig. 1. Overview of the workflow. An unsupervised deformable registration network (*DRN*, top) is combined with *Instance-Specific Optimization (IO)* (bottom) for iterative refinement at test time using the output deformation field of the trained *DRN*. *DRN* as well as *IO* are trained bidirectionally, providing both forward and backward deformation fields. For both modules, the loss function combines either a single or multiple image similarity metrics with a smoothness regularization on the deformation field.

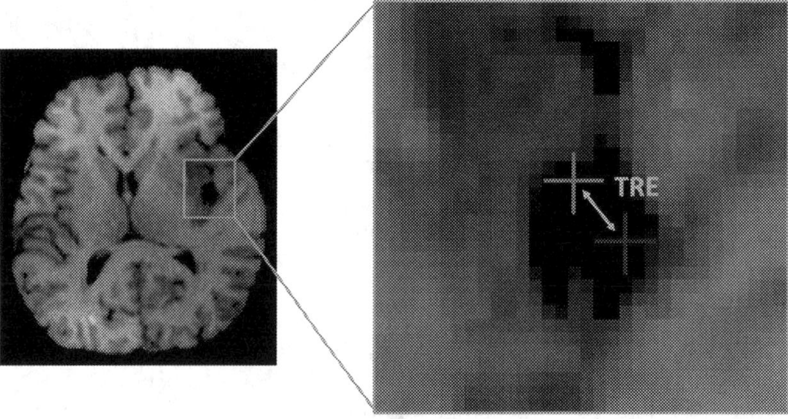

Fig. 2. Illustration of *Target Registration Error (TRE)* evaluation between expert landmark annotation (red) and warped landmark after image registration (blue). The green arrow indicates the Euclidean distance between the two points. For simplicity, the illustration is in 2D, while the actual evaluation is performed in 3D space. (Color figure online)

2.4 Evaluation

We evaluate all experiments by calculating the mean *TRE* between the expert landmark annotations and the warped landmarks on the respective test sets. We use the Euclidean distance to calculate the *TRE*, as illustrated in Fig. 2.

3 Experiments and Results

We perform experiments using different loss functions on two brain *Magnetic Resonance Imaging (MRI)* datasets. Additionally, we implement two reference methods for comparison.

3.1 Data and Pre-processing

Training and evaluation are performed on two brain tumor datasets comprising 419 paired exams in total:

Pre-Post-OP (PP): Contains 300 pairs of brain MR exams with one timepoint before and one timepoint after tumor resection. It is comprised of the official training+validation dataset of *BraTS-Reg* [4] with 160 cases and three datasets collected at *Klinikum rechts der Isar (TUM)* with 49, 30, and 61 cases, respectively.

Pre-Intra-OP (PI): Contains 119 pairs of brain MR exams with one timepoint before and one timepoint during tumor surgery and originates again from *Klinikum rechts der Isar (TUM)*.

Each exam comprises either three or four of the MR sequences *native T1-weighted (T1)*, *T2 Fluid Attenuated Inversion Recovery (FLAIR)*. We preprocess the data using the *BraTS toolkit* [14], which includes reorientation into the same coordinate system, rigid co-registration to a brain atlas as well as brain extraction. Additionally, intensity normalization is applied to all images. For testing, we use 30 cases for *PP* and 20 cases for *PI*. For each test set, six landmarks annotated by clinical experts are provided for each case, accumulating to 180 landmarks on 30 patients for *PP* and 120 landmarks on 20 patients for *PI*.

3.2 Similarity Metrics

We demonstrate the simultaneous optimization strategy on the similarity metrics *MSE* and *NCC*, which are widely used for medical image registration tasks [6].

3.3 Training and Testing

We perform multi-channel training and testing for *DRN* and *IO*. For *PP*, this includes all four sequences, while for *PI*, the sequences *T1*, *T1CE* and *FLAIR* are available. To overcome this imbalance, we train separate networks for *PP* and *PI*. We split the *PP* dataset into training (80%), validation (10%), and test (10%)

and select the model for testing that shows a minimal loss on the validation set. Since we have much fewer cases available for the experiments on the *PI* dataset, we waive the validation set here and decide on a fixed number of 600 training epochs in all experiments. At test time, the *DRN*'s output deformation field serves as input to the 30 iterations of *IO*. For each dataset, we compare the combined loss of *MSE+NCC* against the individual addends, both for the initial *DRN* training as well as the *IO*. Therefore, we exhaustively explore loss combinations for *DRN* and *IO*, as depicted in Table 1.

The implementation is inspired by [6] using *Pytorch* 1.8.1 [20]. We use learning rates 1*e*-4 and 1*e*-3 for *DRN* and *IO*, respectively. Image similarity metrics are weighted equally in the loss function, summing up to 1 for the similarity term. Smoothness regularization weight is set to 1.0 for all experiments for a fair comparison.

3.4 Reference Methods

We compare our approach with two established methods: a deformable *SyN* registration by *ANTs* [3], and *VM* [6], both using the respective T1-weighted sequences. We implement two variants of *VM* [6], available at [5], that employ *MSE* and *NCC* as respective image similarity metrics. Therefore, we use default learning rate 1*e*-4 and recommended smoothness regularization weights of 0.02 and 1.5 for *MSE* and *NCC*, respectively. Likewise, *ANTs SyN* [3] is implemented using default parameters. Since we opt for deformable registration without prior rigid/affine alignment, we apply the same for *VM* and *ANTs SyN*.

Table 1. Mean *TRE* in *mm* with standard deviation using different losses for *DRN* and *DRN+IO* on the Pre-Post-OP and Pre-Intra-OP test sets. Shown are the results on all possible combinations of loss functions. The best result in each category is highlighted. Statistical comparisons are provided in Table 2. Hit rate curves [24] are shown in Fig. 3.

Loss [DRN]	Loss [IO]	Pre-Post-OP	Pre-Intra-OP
MSE	(not applied)	2.40 ± 1.56	3.48 ± 3.45
MSE	MSE	2.21 ± 1.56	3.27 ± 3.46
MSE	NCC	1.81 ± 1.45	3.24 ± 3.39
MSE	MSE+NCC	$\mathbf{1.76 \pm 1.36}$	$\mathbf{3.17 \pm 3.39}$
NCC	(not applied)	2.18 ± 1.52	3.31 ± 2.68
NCC	MSE	2.06 ± 1.50	2.96 ± 2.78
NCC	NCC	1.80 ± 1.44	2.71 ± 2.79
NCC	MSE+NCC	$\mathbf{1.77 \pm 1.36}$	$\mathbf{2.68 \pm 2.72}$
MSE+NCC	(not applied)	2.19 ± 1.49	3.07 ± 2.96
MSE+NCC	MSE	2.07 ± 1.48	2.94 ± 3.05
MSE+NCC	NCC	1.80 ± 1.44	2.86 ± 2.95
MSE+NCC	MSE+NCC	$\mathbf{1.73 \pm 1.34}$	$\mathbf{2.76 \pm 2.89}$

3.5 Results

Table 1 shows quantitative results on both datasets. The *TREs* indicate that for *PP*, *DRN* only with *NCC* loss achieves the lowest mean error. When coupling *DRN* with *IO*, for all possible combinations, mean *TRE* is always lowest when using *MSE+NCC* loss during *IO*. On *PI*, lowest mean *TRE* for *DRN* only is achieved when combining *MSE* and *NCC* in the loss function. When adding *IO*, *DRN* with *NCC* loss coupled with *IO* using *MSE+NCC* loss shows lowest mean *TRE*. Statistical comparisons based on *Paired Samples T-Tests* are provided in Table 2.

Table 2. *P-values* and 95% *Confidence Intervals (CI)* of *Paired Samples T-Tests* on the *TRE* of competitive methods for the Pre-Post-OP and the Pre-Intra-OP datasets. Methods are given by declaring the used losses for *DRN* and *IO*, respectively.

Method 1	Method 2	p-value [CI] (Pre-Post-OP)	p-value [CI] (Pre-Intra-OP)
DRN (NCC)	DRN (MSE+NCC)	0.85 [−0.09; 0.07]	0.05 [0.00; 0.47]
DRN (MSE)+ IO (NCC)	DRN (MSE)+ IO (MSE+NCC)	0.13 [−0.01; 0.10]	0.23 [−0.04; 0.16]
DRN (NCC)+ IO (NCC)	DRN (NCC)+ IO (MSE+NCC)	0.22 [−0.02; 0.08]	0.50 [−0.06; 0.13]
DRN (MSE+NCC)+ IO (NCC)	DRN (MSE+NCC)+ IO (MSE+NCC)	**0.03 [0.01; 0.13]**	**0.03 [0.01; 0.19]**

Table 3. Comparison with reference methods. Mean *TRE* in *mm* with standard deviation on the Pre-Post-OP and Pre-Intra-OP datasets for the best *DRN+IO* compared to *VM* and ANTs *SyN*. The proposed method is on par with established reference registration methods.

Method	Pre-Post-OP	Pre-Intra-OP
DRN+IO	1.73 ± 1.34	2.68 ± 2.72
VM (MSE)	2.98 ± 2.11	3.66 ± 2.90
VM (NCC)	2.09 ± 1.54	2.37 ± 2.37
ANTs SyN	2.02 ± 1.49	1.81 ± 1.17

Moreover, we have evaluated the experiments with respect to their *hit rate* curves according to [24], see Fig. 3, showing the behavior of the different methods with respect to registration accuracy with increased tolerance.

Evaluating performance with respect to running time, we determine that the runtime mainly depends on the implementation of the respective similarity metric. In our case, *NCC* loss is significantly slower than *MSE*. When combining the two metrics in the loss function, there is barely any difference in runtime compared to *NCC* alone, since the runtime of *MSE* is overall negligible. This finding will probably change when the respective implementation differs and/or other similarity metrics are used.

Table 3 shows a comparison of the best *DRN+IO* with results achieved by reference methods *VM* and *ANTs*. For *PP*, *DRN+IO* shows lowest mean *TREs*, while for *PI*, this is the case for *ANTs SyN*.

Our findings are in line with how experts visually perceive the registration quality: In a blinded evaluation of registration methods, three expert radiologists independently picked the *MSE+NCC* registration as their favorite. Asked to provide reasoning for their choice, experts cited better registration quality around ventricles and fewer artifacts, such as unrealistically deformed tissue. Figure 4 shows sample qualitative results on *PI*, illustrating these findings.

4 Discussion

The contribution of this work is to simultaneously optimize multiple image similarity metrics for image registration tasks in a *DL* setting. For demonstration purposes, we combine the well-established metrics *MSE* and *NCC*. We evaluate *DRNs* with and without *IO* in two challenging multi-modal 3D registration settings, namely pre- to post-operative and pre- to intra-operative glioma *MRI*.

Table 1 shows that combining *MSE* and *NCC* losses consistently improves *IO* performance in both datasets. When applied to *DRN* only, the combination still performs best for *PI* while showing comparable results to *NCC* for *PP*. Furthermore, Table 3 illustrates that our method achieves competitive results compared to established reference methods. Moreover, for *PP*, the proposed approach outperforms all reference methods. For *PI*, *ANTs SyN* performs best. A potential explanation might be lower registration quality introduced by the *FLAIR* images. When using *T1* images only for training and testing, the results are getting more comparable, see Table S1 in the supplementary material. Also, *DRN* as well as *VM* would likely benefit from a bigger training dataset. When performing an additional experiment using the Elastix toolbox [13] for single- vs multi-metric registration, we can observe that combining two metrics improves performance for *PI*, see Table S2 in the supplementary material.

Combining *MSE* and *NCC* can help to improve the alignment of the source image to the target image. The qualitative assessment by clinical experts supports these findings.

There are several limitations to this study. The evaluation is performed on rather small test sets of 20 for *PI* and 30 for *PP*. The used datasets are fairly specific, so for generalization purposes, an extension toward other registration tasks promises to yield additional insights. Here, we focus on multi-sequence training on all available MR sequences using a 4D implementation of the *NCC* loss. Training on different sequences separately will possibly indicate increased understanding on the respective influences. Performing cross validation for model

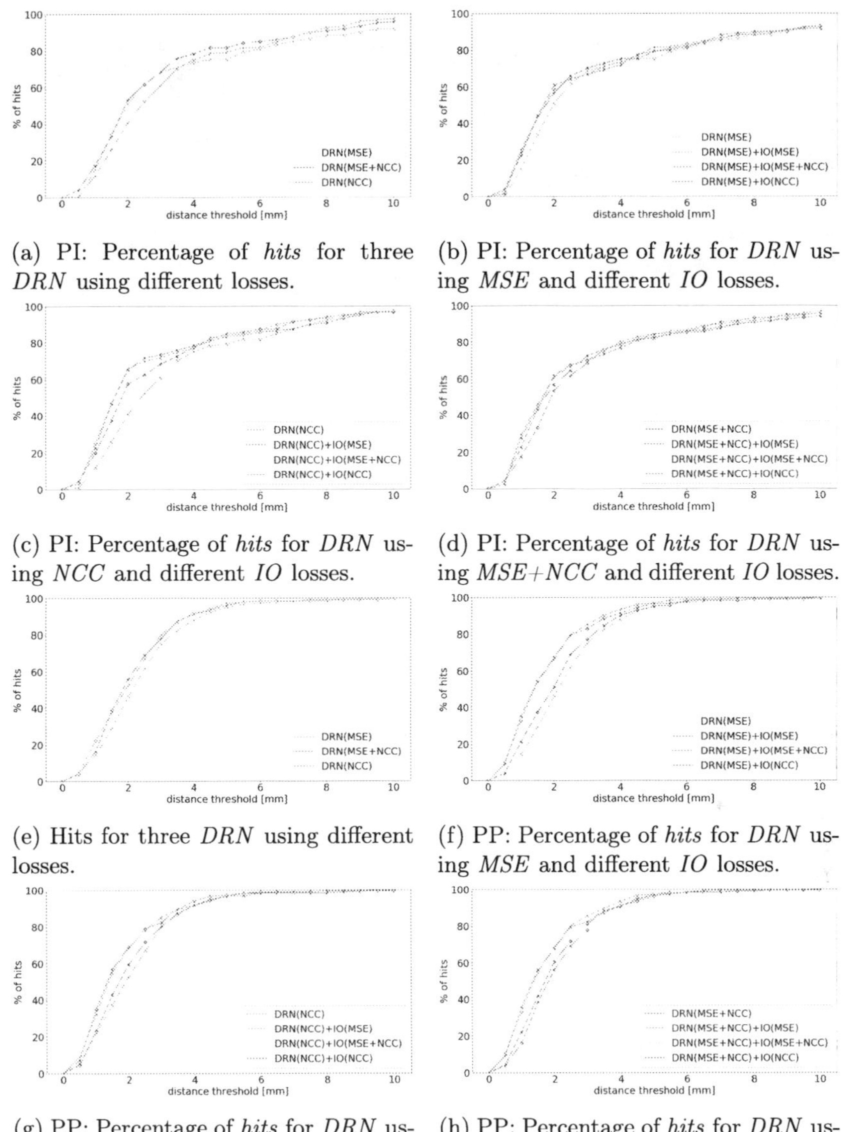

(a) PI: Percentage of *hits* for three *DRN* using different losses.

(b) PI: Percentage of *hits* for *DRN* using *MSE* and different *IO* losses.

(c) PI: Percentage of *hits* for *DRN* using *NCC* and different *IO* losses.

(d) PI: Percentage of *hits* for *DRN* using *MSE+NCC* and different *IO* losses.

(e) Hits for three *DRN* using different losses.

(f) PP: Percentage of *hits* for *DRN* using *MSE* and different *IO* losses.

(g) PP: Percentage of *hits* for *DRN* using *NCC* and different *IO* losses.

(h) PP: Percentage of *hits* for *DRN* using *MSE+NCC* and different *IO* losses.

Fig. 3. Hit rate curves [24] on PI and PP, respectively. *Hit* denotes that a warped landmark lies within a certain distance threshold to the respective expert landmark annotation. Here, evaluation thresholds are set every $0.5mm$, *hit* percentages in between are interpolated.

selection might improve stability in the results. Even though the regularization could be fine-tuned, we use a fixed weight on the deformation field in our approach.

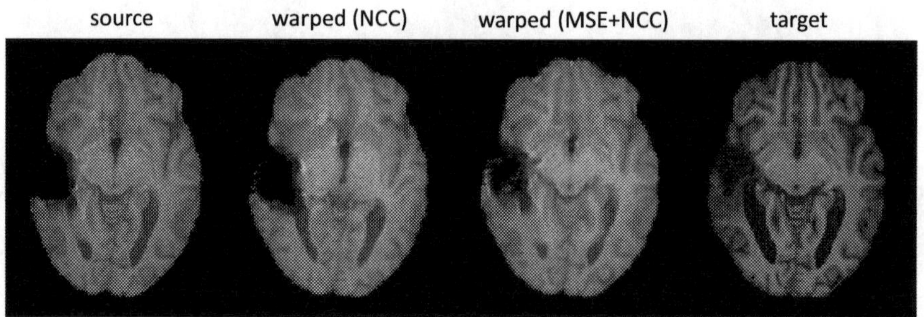

Fig. 4. Sample registration results on the Pre-Intra-OP dataset. Registration with combined losses *MSE+NCC* shows improved registration in comparison to registration with *NCC* only, especially nearby the tumor and the resection cavity, respectively.

5 Conclusion and Future Work

We propose an optimization strategy – here implemented by means of a simple summation – that benefits registration performance with regard to *TRE*. Moreover, we conduct extensive comparisons against established reference methods. Future work should investigate the addition of further similarity metrics such as *Mutual Information*. Besides, introducing different weights for the individual parts of the loss function (instead of equally weighting) might further enhance registration performance.

Acknowledgements. Supported by Deutsche Forschungsgemeinschaft (DFG) through TUM International Graduate School of Science and Engineering (IGSSE), GSC 81. BM, BW and FK are supported through the SFB 824, subproject B12. BM acknowledges support by the Helmut Horten Foundation. Finally, we acknowledge Andreas Poschenrieder and Anna Valentina Lioba Eleonora Claire Javid Mamasani for eye-opening insights.

References

1. Avants, B., et al.: Multivariate analysis of structural and diffusion imaging in traumatic brain injury. Acad. Radiol. **15**(11), 1360–1375 (2008)
2. Avants, B.B., Tustison, N.J., Song, G., Cook, P.A., Klein, A., Gee, J.C.: A reproducible evaluation of ants similarity metric performance in brain image registration. Neuroimage **54**(3), 2033–2044 (2011)
3. Avants, B.B., Tustison, N., Song, G., et al.: Advanced normalization tools (ANTS). Insight J. **2**(365), 1–35 (2009)
4. Baheti, B., et al.: The brain tumor sequence registration challenge: establishing correspondence between pre-operative and follow-up MRI scans of diffuse glioma patients. arXiv preprint arXiv:2112.06979 (2021)
5. Balakrishnan, G., Zhao, A., Sabuncu, M., Guttag, J., Dalca, A.V.: voxelmorph: learning-based image registration. https://github.com/voxelmorph/voxelmorph

6. Balakrishnan, G., Zhao, A., Sabuncu, M.R., Guttag, J., Dalca, A.V.: Voxelmorph: a learning framework for deformable medical image registration. IEEE Trans. Med. Imaging **38**(8), 1788–1800 (2019)
7. Boukellouz, W., Moussaoui, A.: Evaluation of several similarity measures for deformable image registration using T1-weighted MR images of the brain. In: 2017 5th International Conference on Electrical Engineering-Boumerdes (ICEE-B), pp. 1–5. IEEE (2017)
8. Canalini, L., Klein, J., Gerken, A., Heldmann, S., Hering, A., Hahn, H.K.: Iterative method to register longitudinal MRI acquisitions in neurosurgical context. In: Brainlesion: Glioma, Multiple Sclerosis, Stroke and Traumatic Brain Injuries, pp. 262–272. Springer, Cham (2023)
9. Chen, J., Frey, E.C., He, Y., Segars, W.P., Li, Y., Du, Y.: Transmorph: transformer for unsupervised medical image registration. Med. Image Anal. **82**, 102615 (2022)
10. Ferrante, E., Dokania, P.K., Marini, R., Paragios, N.: Deformable registration through learning of context-specific metric aggregation. In: Wang, Q., Shi, Y., Suk, H.-I., Suzuki, K. (eds.) MLMI 2017. LNCS, vol. 10541, pp. 256–265. Springer, Cham (2017). https://doi.org/10.1007/978-3-319-67389-9_30
11. Fidon, L., et al.: A dempster-shafer approach to trustworthy AI with application to fetal brain MRI segmentation. arXiv preprint arXiv:2204.02779 (2022)
12. Großbröhmer, C., Siebert, H., Hansen, L., Heinrich, M.P.: Employing convexadam for brats-reg. In: Brainlesion: Glioma, Multiple Sclerosis, Stroke and Traumatic Brain Injuries, pp. 252–261. Springer, Cham (2023)
13. Klein, S., Staring, M., Murphy, K., Viergever, M.A., Pluim, J.P.: Elastix: a toolbox for intensity-based medical image registration. IEEE Trans. Med. Imaging **29**(1), 196–205 (2009)
14. Kofler, F., et al.: Brats toolkit: translating brats brain tumor segmentation algorithms into clinical and scientific practice. Front. Neurosci. 125 (2020)
15. Kofler, F., et al.: Are we using appropriate segmentation metrics? Identifying correlates of human expert perception for CNN training beyond rolling the dice coefficient. Mach. Learn. Biomed. Imaging **2**(May 2023 issue), 27–71 (2023)
16. Kofler, F., et al.: blob loss: instance imbalance aware loss functions for semantic segmentation. In: International Conference on Information Processing in Medical Imaging, pp. 755–767. Springer, Cham (2023)
17. Meng, M., Bi, L., Feng, D., Kim, J.: Brain tumor sequence registration with non-iterative coarse-to-fine networks and dual deep supervision. In: Brainlesion: Glioma, Multiple Sclerosis, Stroke and Traumatic Brain Injuries, pp. 273–282. Springer, Cham (2023)
18. Mok, T.C., Chung, A.: Robust image registration with absent correspondences in pre-operative and follow-up brain MRI scans of diffuse glioma patients. In: Brainlesion: Glioma, Multiple Sclerosis, Stroke and Traumatic Brain Injuries, pp. 231–240. Springer, Cham (2023)
19. Mok, T.C.W., Chung, A.C.S.: Large deformation diffeomorphic image registration with laplacian pyramid networks. In: Martel, A.L., et al. (eds.) MICCAI 2020. LNCS, vol. 12263, pp. 211–221. Springer, Cham (2020). https://doi.org/10.1007/978-3-030-59716-0_21
20. Paszke, A., et al.: PyTorch: an imperative style, high-performance deep learning library. In: Wallach, H., Larochelle, H., Beygelzimer, A., d'Alché Buc, F., Fox, E., Garnett, R. (eds.) Advances in Neural Information Processing Systems 32, pp. 8024–8035. Curran Associates, Inc. (2019). http://papers.neurips.cc/paper/9015-pytorch-an-imperative-style-high-performance-deep-learning-library.pdf

21. Rueckert, D., Sonoda, L.I., Hayes, C., Hill, D.L., Leach, M.O., Hawkes, D.J.: Non-rigid registration using free-form deformations: application to breast MR images. IEEE Trans. Med. Imaging **18**(8), 712–721 (1999)
22. Uss, M.L., Vozel, B., Abramov, S.K., Chehdi, K.: Selection of a similarity measure combination for a wide range of multimodal image registration cases. IEEE Trans. Geosci. Remote Sens. **59**(1), 60–75 (2020)
23. Wachs, J., Stern, H., Burks, T., Alchanatis, V.: Multi-modal registration using a combined similarity measure. Appl. Soft Comput. **52**, 159–168 (2009)
24. Waldmannstetter, D., et al.: Framing image registration as a landmark detection problem for better representation of clinical relevance. arXiv preprint arXiv:2308.01318 (2023)
25. Wodzinski, M., Jurgas, A., Marini, N., Atzori, M., Müller, H.: Unsupervised method for intra-patient registration of brain magnetic resonance images based on objective function weighting by inverse consistency: Contribution to the brats-reg challenge. In: Brainlesion: Glioma, Multiple Sclerosis, Stroke and Traumatic Brain Injuries, pp. 241–251. Springer, Cham (2023)
26. Zhou, J., Liu, Q.: A combined similarity measure for multimodal image registration. In: 2015 IEEE International Conference on Imaging Systems and Techniques (IST), pp. 1–5. IEEE (2015)

ReFuSeg: Regularized Multi-modal Fusion for Precise Brain Tumour Segmentation

Aditya Kasliwal[1(✉)], Sankarshanaa Sagaram[1], Laven Srivastava[2], Pratinav Seth[1], and Adil Khan[3]

[1] Department of Data Science and Computer Applications, Manipal Institute of Technology, Manipal Academy of Higher Education, Manipal, India
kasliwaladitya17@gmail.com

[2] Department of Computer Science, Manipal Institute of Technology, Manipal Academy of Higher Education, Manipal, India

[3] Department of Mechanical Engineering, Manipal Institute of Technology, Manipal Academy of Higher Education, Manipal, India

Abstract. Semantic segmentation of brain tumours is a fundamental task in medical image analysis that can help clinicians in diagnosing the patient and tracking the progression of any malignant entities. Accurate segmentation of brain lesions is essential for medical diagnosis and treatment planning. However, failure to acquire specific MRI imaging modalities can prevent applications from operating in critical situations, raising concerns about their reliability and overall trustworthiness. This paper presents a novel multi-modal approach for brain lesion segmentation that leverages information from four distinct imaging modalities while being robust to real-world scenarios of missing modalities, such as T1, T1c, T2, and FLAIR MRI of brains. Our proposed method can help address the challenges posed by artifacts in medical imagery due to data acquisition errors (such as patient motion) or a reconstruction algorithm's inability to represent the anatomy while ensuring a trade-off in accuracy. Our proposed regularization module makes it robust to these scenarios and ensures the reliability of lesion segmentation.

Keywords: Brain Lesion · Multi-modality Segmentation · Missing Modality Learning

1 Introduction

The rise of Artificial Intelligence in healthcare has made AI-based interventions for brain tumour diagnosis and pre-assessment increasingly vital. Analyzing brain tumours through AI-driven techniques contributes significantly and helps in understanding the progression of brain tumour cells and assisting in surgical groundwork. Characterization of these segmented tumours can directly aid in predicting the interim duration for diagnosis and the patient's overall

S. Sagaram and L. Srivastava—Authors have contributed equally.

U. Baid et al. (Eds.): BrainLes 2023/SWITCH 2023, LNCS 14668, pp. 69–80, 2024.
https://doi.org/10.1007/978-3-031-76160-7_7

life expectancy, making brain tumour segmentation crucial for various applications in this field. Magnetic Resonance Imaging (MRI) is a reliable diagnostic tool that is crucial in monitoring and planning brain tumour surgeries. The recent advancements in automated brain tumour segmentation using MRI have achieved remarkable success and practical utility. [5,19] These algorithms typically rely on multiple modalities, with the four most relevant being T1-weighted images with and without contrast enhancement, T2-weighted images, and FLAIR images. Combining these complementary 3D MRI modalities, such as T1, T1 with contrast agent (T1c), T2, and Fluid-attenuated Inversion Recovery (FLAIR), helps highlight different tissue properties and regions where the tumour has spread. The integration of multiple modalities is essential for capturing a comprehensive view of the brain and improving segmentation accuracy. Each modality provides unique insights into the underlying tissue properties and pathology, allowing the model to exploit complementary information for robust and precise lesion segmentation.

While deep learning-based brain tumour segmentation techniques have shown impressive performance in various benchmarks, they face challenges due to the limited kernel size in typical image segmentation models [7,19]. This limitation hinders their ability to learn long-range dependencies necessary for accurately segmenting tumours of various shapes and sizes. In clinical routines, missing MRI sequences due to time constraints or image artifacts can be a common challenge. Therefore, developing methods that can compensate for missing modalities and recover segmentation performance is highly desirable, promoting the broader adoption of these algorithms in clinical practice.

We propose ReFuSeg: Regularized Multi-Modal Fusion for Precise Brain Lesion Segmentation, our proposed architecture utilizes a novel approach toward contrastive regularisation to learn features between multiple modalities. Our approach prevents the model from overfitting to any particular modality and promotes the learning of complementary information from each modality.

This leads to more robust and generalizable features capable of capturing the intrinsic characteristics of each modality. All four encoders work independently, learning individual features amongst each modality which helps it maintain robustness within its predictions as it is not dependent on any one singular modality to make accurate segmentation predictions.

The effectiveness of our proposed approach has been validated through experimental evaluations on the BraTS 23 dataset [1,2,16]. Our method displays robustness in accurately segmenting brain lesions, even in the case of missing modalities where they exhibit outstanding Dice and Hausdorff-95 scores, even when provided with only limited portions of the original data. Furthermore, the proposed model is unaffected by the inclusion of noise artifacts, which are commonly found in everyday clinical usage. Owing to these promising results, we demonstrate the suitability of our approach for real-world scenarios.

2 Related Works

2.1 Multimodal Image Segmentation

Previous methodologies have explored various approaches to address the segmentation challenge. Some studies have incorporated 3D network convolutions which fused the correlation representations via attention guided mechanisms [26]. A distinct approach was taken by Havaei et al. [6], where they constructed a unified model through a self-supervised training pipeline for each channel. Instead of using volumetric data, they directly passed 2D slices into the model encoders. Predictions from multiple channels were combined by merging feature maps, and mean, and variance were computed to achieve the final segmentation. In another study [22], a cascaded network [14] was employed. In the first stage, the tumour was segmented, and subsequent stages focused on learning substructures for more detailed segmentation.

2.2 Missing Modalities

A popular technique [4] involves utilizing an adversarial loss on intermediate feature maps from two domains, facilitating knowledge transfer between these domains. Similarly, in a different work [15], a class-specific adversarial loss was employed on feature maps to transfer a learned network from a source domain to a target domain. Generative models [24] have also been used in the past to synthesize missing modalities. Furthermore, self-supervised learning techniques have been utilized [21] by randomly dropping modalities during training and leveraging the learned combined feature maps. These feature maps are then adjusted to match any encoder distributions to compensate for the missing data.

2.3 Contrastive Learning

A powerful mechanism for representation learning is contrastive learning. The core principle involves training a neural network to map similar inputs closer together in a learned feature space while simultaneously pushing dissimilar inputs further apart. [3] Contrastive loss minimizes dissimilarity between positive examples based on the learned features. Contrastive learning enables the effective learning of shared and discriminative representations across these modalities by capitalizing on the inherent similarities and distinctions across different modalities. A combination of inter and intra-modal feature learning [23]has also been used to capture similarities and minimize disagreement between each modality. In biomedical segmentation, [13] a network was proposed where one encoder learns features from T1 modality while the secondary segmentation backbone consisting of Convolution blocks takes in the multi-modal images and minimizes contrastive loss.

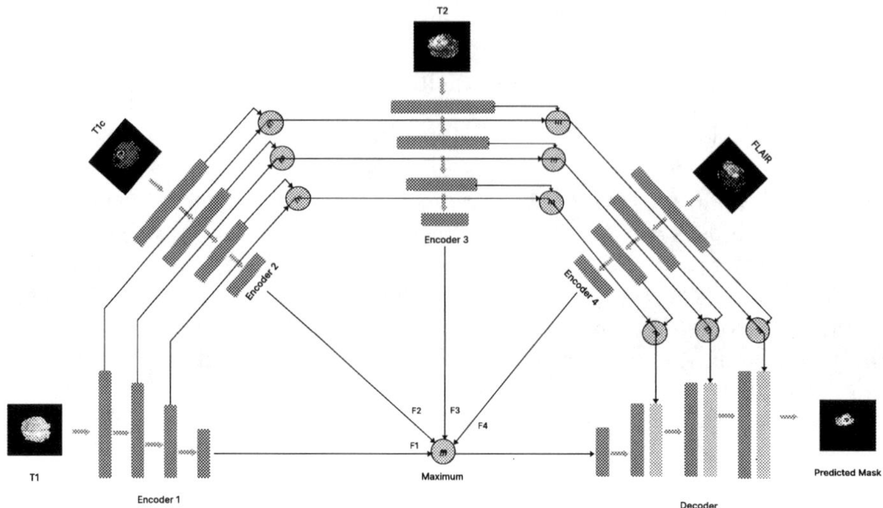

Fig. 1. Proposed ReFuSeg architecture for brain tumour segmentation. The red arrows depict Convolution layers, while the blue boxes show downsampling of extracted features. The element-wise maximum of 4 encoders is then taken, which is passed on to the decoder layer.(Color figure online)

3 Methodology

In this paper, we introduce a novel methodology for brain lesion segmentation which is robust in the case of missing modalities due to the independent working of all the encoders, as a solution for the BraTS 2023 Adult Glioma Segmentation challenge [2,17] which involves generating segmented tumour masks by utilizing the four modalities provided in the dataset for each instance, i.e., T1, T1 with contrast agent (T1c), T2 and Fluid-attenuated Inversion Recovery (FLAIR). Our proposed approach, illustrated in the figures, comprises two primary components:

1. A multi-modal U-Net [20] based architecture incorporating four ResNet-34 [11] encoders alongside a feature fusion technique.
2. A regularization module that receives final features from the four encoders, after which contrastive loss is calculated in the backward pass, enabling robustness in case of missing modality.

For our encoders, we use the vastly popular U-net. We make use of four individual encoders for each modality, which progressively down-samples the input image through convolutional and max-pooling layers, capturing features at varying levels of abstraction. In an adapted version featuring four distinct encoders, each is designed to pinpoint particular attributes with each MRI modality. The decoder subsequently enlarges these attributes using transpose convolution techniques, while bridging links from the encoder guarantees the merging of both intricate and broad image nuances. This specialized configuration equips U-Net

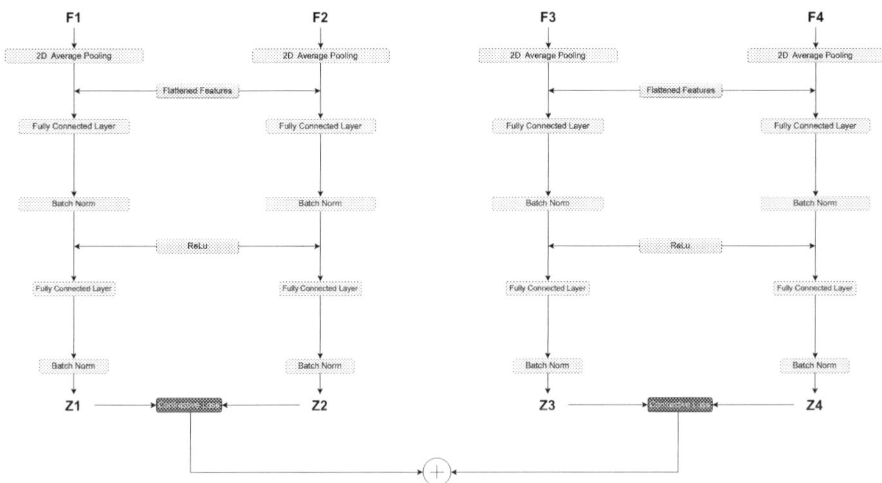

Fig. 2. Computing the final pair-wise losses using the final feature maps of each of the four encoders. Contrastive loss is calculated independently in pairs of 2 each, which is then added to obtain the final contrastive loss.

to adeptly manage spatial complexities in images, positioning it as a prime choice for tasks such as feature extraction.

3.1 Contrastive Regularization

In our proposed approach, the features extracted from the encoders are directed to four distinct contrastive modules. As shown in Fig. 2, each contrastive module comprises a series of layers, including average pooling, fully connected, and batch normalization, followed by another fully connected layer and batch normalization. The resulting outputs from these contrastive modules are instrumental in calculating the contrastive loss similar to the approach used in [8], which is then added to our final loss function. Notably, the T1 and T1c modalities have a higher likelihood of containing similar features due to the nature of their MRI image acquisition methods, i.e., the feature changes noticeable in both modalities are primarily made in the post-processing of the MRI scans; the same is true for T2 and FLAIR modalities. However, the learning process is unaffected by redundant features because contrastive loss is a regularizing mechanism for these modalities. It promotes efficient selection of features and enhances individual contributions during the learning process.

3.2 Feature Transfer from Encoders to Decoder

Once the features are extracted from all four encoders, a new feature map is generated by taking the element-wise maximum of the corresponding level feature maps from each encoder. This ensures that the most relevant features from each encoder are selected, resulting in a new feature map that effectively captures pertinent information from all modalities. The decoder, which comprises several decoding blocks, then receives the new feature map through skip connections. During the upsampling process, the decoder combines these upsampled feature maps with their corresponding counterparts from the encoders, utilizing the skip connections. However, in this modified U-Net model, the skip connections transfer the newly calculated feature map from the four encoders rather than individual feature maps from each encoder. By amalgamating features extracted from the T1, T1c, T2, and FLAIR MRI images across multiple levels of abstraction, the adapted U-Net model demonstrates its capability to generate high-quality outputs.

3.3 Handling Missing Modalities

When faced with missing modalities, such as the absence of a T1-weighted scan in the input, our model exhibits robust performance due to the independent functioning of the four encoders. The model effectively utilizes the available encoders corresponding to the present modalities in such situations. The multilevel feature maps extracted from these encoders are directly passed to the decoder via the skip connections. This approach ensures the model can still capture relevant features from the available input data and produce accurate outputs, even in missing modalities.

3.4 Loss Function

Dice Loss. The Dice loss [18] serves as a metric to assess the overlap between binary predicted and ground truth masks in image segmentation tasks. Its objective is to maximize the similarity between these masks. Therefore, minimizing the Dice loss during model training leads to improved accuracy of the segmentation model. Additionally, our experiments demonstrate that combining Dice loss with contrastive loss further enhances the segmentation performance.

$$\text{Dice Loss} = 1 - \frac{2\sum_{i=1}^{n} y_i \hat{y} i}{\sum_{i=1}^{n} y_i^2 + \sum_{i=1}^{n} \hat{y}_i^2} \tag{1}$$

where y_i represents the ground truth value for the i-th sample, and $\hat{y}_i$ represents the corresponding predicted value from the model. The summation runs over all n samples in the dataset.

Focal Loss. The Focal loss [12] introduces a modulating term to the cross-entropy [25] loss, aiming to prioritize learning on challenging misclassified examples. This dynamic scaling of the cross entropy loss involves the scaling factor diminishing to zero as confidence in the correct class rises. In the context of image segmentation tasks, the Focal loss assumes a pivotal role in handling class imbalance and accentuating challenging samples, resulting in notable improvements in segmentation performance. The Focal loss formula is given as follows:

$$\text{Focal Loss} = -\frac{1}{n}\sum_{i=1}^{n}(\alpha(1-\hat{y}_i)^{\gamma} y_i \log(\hat{y}_i) + (1-\alpha)\hat{y}_i^{\gamma}(1-y_i)\log(1-\hat{y}_i)) \tag{2}$$

In the formula, y_i represents the ground truth value (0 or 1) for the i-th sample, and $\hat{y}_i$ represents the corresponding predicted value from the model. The summation runs over all n samples in the dataset.

The adjustable hyperparameters, α and γ, enable us to control the focusing effect and the rate at which the loss decreases for well-classified samples. Integrating the Focal loss with other appropriate loss functions, such as the contrastive loss mentioned in our experiments, can improve segmentation results.

Contrastive Loss. Contrastive loss [9] serves as a fundamental loss function utilized in machine learning to train models for similarity learning. Its purpose is to facilitate learning data representations, wherein similar data points are brought closer together in the representation space while dissimilar data points are pushed further apart. This enhances image fidelity and realism by reducing artifacts and noise in the output images. In their work, [3] applied this contrastive loss to train their model by comparing pairs of images and calculating a similarity score between them. The contrastive loss formula is defined as follows:

$$l(v_i, v_j) = -\log\left(\frac{\exp(\text{sim}(v_i, v_j))}{\sum_{k \neq i} \exp(\text{sim}(v_i, v_k))}\right) \tag{3}$$

Here, v_i and v_j represent the representations of two modalities of the same instance and sim(,) denotes the function computing the cosine similarity. The denominator in the formula represents the sum over all views k in the batch, excluding i. Subsequently, the contrastive loss is computed over the corresponding instances of two modalities in the batch of size N and is then averaged as:

$$L_C = \frac{1}{2N}\sum_{i=1}^{N}\left[l(v_{\text{ix}}, v_{\text{iy}}) + l(v_{\text{iy}}, v_{\text{ix}})\right] \tag{4}$$

$$\forall\,(x, y) = [(T1, T1c), (T2, FLAIR)]$$

The resulting L_C contributes to the overall loss function, which is critical in guiding the model's training process for similarity learning and image representation enhancement.

Final Loss. The final loss employed in our paper, achieved after rigorous evaluation of different hyperparameter combinations, is represented as follows:

$$L_{Final} = 0.5 \cdot L_{Dice} + 0.5 \cdot L_{Focal} + \beta \cdot L_C \tag{5}$$

Here, β acts as a switch for contrastive loss in the overall loss function.

4 Experimental Analysis

The BraTS [1,2,17], 2023 dataset was used in our study, which consisted of 5,880 MRI scans from 1,470 patients with brain diffuse glioma. The BraTS mpMRI scans were provided in NIfTI format (.nii.gz) and included native (T1) and post-contrast T1-weighted (T1c), T2-weighted (T2), and T2 Fluid Attenuated Inversion Recovery (FLAIR) volumes. The training dataset had 1,251 instances,

Table 1. Validation Results for BraTS 2023 Dataset.

Contrastive	Dice			Hausdorff		
Regularisation	ET	TC	WT	ET	TC	WT
×	0.792	0.828	0.909	22.9	14.07	7.34
✓	0.786	0.832	0.910	21.8	9.17	7.08

while the validation dataset had 219 instances. We submitted our predicted results on the validation dataset to the challenge website to assess our model's performance.

The original 3D files, each of size $240 \times 240 \times 155$, were preprocessed into 155 2D slices of dimensionality 240×240. This preprocessing step addressed spatial invariance, reduced computational complexity, and enhanced anatomical interpretability. Additionally, we applied several augmentations to the data, including horizontal and vertical flips with probabilities of 0.5, rotation with a limit of 20°C, shift limit of 0.1, and probability of 0.5, random crop to a size of 224×224, and final resizing to 240×240.

We used softmax as the activation function in the output layer. The performance of the model was evaluated using the Dice score and Hausdorff-95 distance. The Dice score is a metric that measures the overlap between two sets, and a high Dice score indicates that the model has accurately captured the boundaries and shapes of the target structure. The Hausdorff-95 distance, on the other hand, measures the distance between the nearest points of two sets, and it is specifically used to assess the model's performance at boundary regions. To comprehensively evaluate the model, both these metrics were employed in our analysis. Our model was trained using the Adam optimizer [10] with a learning rate of 10^{-4}. During the initial experimentation, the proposed model was trained for 50 epochs without contrastive regularization. Subsequently, another training run was conducted with contrastive regularization. The comparison of results between non-contrastive and contrastive regularization can be found in Table 1.

To evaluate the model's robustness when faced with missing modalities, we performed inference four times, each time excluding one of the four available modalities. We conducted this inference process for both non-contrastive and contrastive approaches, and the detailed results are presented in Table 2.

5 Results

The validation results, reveal noteworthy insights into the impact of contrastive regularization on the model's performance. As shown in Table 1, these findings demonstrate a remarkable and favorable improvement in the model's performance when contrastive regularization is employed, in comparison to its performance without this technique.

As indicated in Table 1, the model exhibited signs of overfitting on specific modalities when contrastive regularization was not utilized. In such cases, the

Table 2. Comparing impact of missing modalities on BraTS 2023 validation set, with and without contrastive regularization.

Modality	Contrastive	Dice			Hausdorff-95		
Dropped	Regularisation	ET	TC	WT	ET	TC	WT
T1	×	0.753	0.824	0.901	40.01	17.76	14.18
T1	✓	**0.769**	**0.833**	**0.908**	**31.04**	**13.26**	**9.59**
T1c	×	0.074	0.322	**0.878**	253.92	45.08	**11.47**
T1c	✓	**0.762**	**0.803**	0.874	**38.91**	**22.06**	30.83
T2	×	0.057	0.271	0.884	200.89	65.63	**7.17**
T2	✓	**0.783**	**0.819**	**0.89**	**27.41**	**17.5**	16.22
FLAIR	×	0.745	0.703	0.401	38.00	26.85	27.96
FLAIR	✓	**0.768**	**0.786**	**0.524**	**27.01**	**23.56**	**21.97**

model excessively relied on a limited subset of the available modalities. As a result, the model's overall performance suffered significantly during validation, especially when confronted with missing modalities. Conversely, incorporating contrastive regularization yielded substantial enhancement in the model's performance in the presence of missing modalities, demonstrating reduced reliance on any single modality (T1, T1c, T2, or T2 flair) and, instead, effectively harnessing features from all available modalities. This regularization effect signifies the model's adept utilization of features across all modalities, effectively mitigating the overfitting challenges.

6 Conclusion

This research paper introduces a novel framework that integrates data fusion and regularization techniques for semantic segmentation, utilizing four encoders within a U-Net-based architecture. The proposed framework serves as our response to the BraTS 2023 Adult Glioma Segmentation challenge [1,2,17], held at the 9th MICCAI Workshop on Brain Lesions (BrainLes). It represents a straightforward and resource-efficient architecture compared to other models in this field.

Our architecture yields outstanding results with Dice scores of 0.786, 0.832, and 0.910, as well as Hausdorff distances of 21.8, 9.17, and 7.08 for the enhancing tumour (ET), tumour core (TC), and whole tumour (WT) classes respectively, on the validation dataset with contrastive regularization. The model possesses the ability to be robust in handling missing data and maintaining its efficacy even when dealing with absent modalities, as demonstrated in Table 2. Notably, we believe to be the first to present such a fusion model that effectively addresses missing modalities, rendering our architecture highly suitable for real-world scenarios with frequently occurring missing data.

Our research addresses challenges in semantic segmentation and offers opportunities for improved performance and broader use. We plan to move from a 2D approach to a 3D U-Net structure, considering the volume-based nature of medical imaging. We also intend to test our model under different noisy conditions to assess its robustness in real-world clinical scenarios.

We are eager to explore further experiments involving the scaling of contrastive regularization as well as investigating the applicability of this approach in diverse domains and industries, broadening its potential impact. We aim to apply our approach not only to brain tumors but also to other areas like cardiology and orthopedics. Another focus will be integrating attention mechanisms, which could help the model emphasize important image areas. By adding a time-based view, we hope to evolve from just diagnosis to ongoing monitoring, tracking tumor development and treatment results. We are driven to develop a model that bridges academic insights with practical clinical use.

Acknowledgments. We would like to thank Mars Rover Manipal, an interdisciplinary student project team of MAHE, for providing the necessary resources for our research. We are grateful to our faculty advisor, Dr Ujjwal Verma, for providing the necessary guidance.

References

1. Baid, U., et al.: The RSNA-ASNR-MICCAI BraTS 2021 benchmark on brain tumor segmentation and radiogenomic classification. ArXiv **abs/2107.02314** (2021). https://api.semanticscholar.org/CorpusID:235742974
2. Bakas, S., et al.: Advancing the cancer genome atlas glioma mri collections with expert segmentation labels and radiomic features. Sci. Data **4** (2017). https://api.semanticscholar.org/CorpusID:3697707
3. Chen, T., Kornblith, S., Norouzi, M., Hinton, G.: A simple framework for contrastive learning of visual representations. In: International Conference on Machine Learning, pp. 1597–1607. PMLR (2020)
4. Ganin, Y., Lempitsky, V.: Unsupervised domain adaptation by backpropagation. In: International Conference on Machine Learning, pp. 1180–1189. PMLR (2015)
5. Grover, V., Tognarelli, J., Crossey, M., Cox, I., Taylor-Robinson, S., McPhail, M.: Magnetic resonance imaging: principles and techniques: Lessons for clinicians. J. Clin. Exper. Hepatol. **5** (2015). https://doi.org/10.1016/j.jceh.2015.08.001
6. Havaei, M., et al.: Brain tumor segmentation with deep neural networks. Med. Image Anal. **35**, 18–31 (2017)
7. Kamnitsas, K., et al.: Ensembles of multiple models and architectures for robust brain tumour segmentation. CoRR **abs/1711.01468** (2017). http://arxiv.org/abs/1711.01468
8. Kasliwal, A., Seth, P., Rallabandi, S.: Corefusion: contrastive regularized fusion for guided thermal super-resolution. 2023 IEEE/CVF Conference on Computer Vision and Pattern Recognition Workshops (CVPRW), pp. 507–514 (2023). https://api.semanticscholar.org/CorpusID:257921158

9. Khosla, P., et al.: Supervised contrastive learning. Adv. Neural. Inf. Process. Syst. **33**, 18661–18673 (2020)
10. Kingma, D.P., Ba, J.: Adam: a method for stochastic optimization. arXiv preprint arXiv:1412.6980 (2014)
11. Koonce, B., Koonce, B.: Resnet 34. Convolutional neural networks with swift for Tensorflow: image recognition and dataset categorization, pp. 51–61 (2021)
12. Lin, T., Goyal, P., Girshick, R.B., He, K., Dollár, P.: Focal loss for dense object detection. CoRR **abs/1708.02002** (2017). http://arxiv.org/abs/1708.02002
13. Liu, H., Nie, D., Shen, D., Wang, J., Tang, Z.: Multimodal brain tumor segmentation using contrastive learning based feature comparison with monomodal normal brain images. In: Wang, L., Dou, Q., Fletcher, P.T., Speidel, S., Li, S. (eds.) Medical Image Computing and Computer Assisted Intervention - MICCAI 2022, pp. 118–127. Springer Nature Switzerland, Cham (2022)
14. Malmi, E., Parambath, S., Peyrat, J.M., Abinahed, J., Chawla, S.: Cabs: a cascaded brain tumor segmentation approach, pp. 42–47. Proceedings MICCAI Brain, Tumor Segmentation (BRATS) (2015)
15. Manders, J., van Laarhoven, T., Marchiori, E.: Adversarial alignment of class prediction uncertainties for domain adaptation. arXiv preprint arXiv:1804.04448 (2018)
16. Menze, B.H., et al.: The multimodal brain tumor image segmentation benchmark (brats). IEEE Trans. Med. Imaging **34**(10), 1993–2024 (2015). https://doi.org/10.1109/TMI.2014.2377694
17. Menze, B.H., et al.: The multimodal brain tumor image segmentation benchmark (brats). IEEE Trans. Med. Imaging **34**, 1993–2024 (2015). https://api.semanticscholar.org/CorpusID:1739295
18. Milletari, F., Navab, N., Ahmadi, S.: V-net: fully convolutional neural networks for volumetric medical image segmentation. CoRR **abs/1606.04797** (2016). http://arxiv.org/abs/1606.04797
19. Myronenko, A.: 3d MRI brain tumor segmentation using autoencoder regularization. CoRR **abs/1810.11654** (2018). http://arxiv.org/abs/1810.11654
20. Ronneberger, O., Fischer, P., Brox, T.: U-net: convolutional networks for biomedical image segmentation. In: Medical Image Computing and Computer-Assisted Intervention–MICCAI 2015: 18th International Conference, Munich, Germany, 5-9 October 2015, Proceedings, Part III 18, pp. 234–241. Springer (2015)
21. Shen, Y., Gao, M.: Brain tumor segmentation on mri with missing modalities. In: Chung, A.C.S., Gee, J.C., Yushkevich, P.A., Bao, S. (eds.) Information Processing in Medical Imaging, pp. 417–428. Springer International Publishing, Cham (2019)
22. Wang, G., Li, W., Ourselin, S., Vercauteren, T.: Automatic brain tumor segmentation based on cascaded convolutional neural networks with uncertainty estimation. Front. Comput. Neurosci. **13** (2019). https://doi.org/10.3389/fncom.2019.00056, https://www.frontiersin.org/articles/10.3389/fncom.2019.00056
23. Yuan, X., et al.: Multimodal contrastive training for visual representation learning. In: Proceedings of the IEEE/CVF Conference on Computer Vision and Pattern Recognition, pp. 6995–7004 (2021)
24. Zhang, Y., Brady, M., Smith, S.M.: Segmentation of brain mr images through a hidden markov random field model and the expectation-maximization algorithm. IEEE Trans. Med. Imaging **20**, 45–57 (2001). https://api.semanticscholar.org/CorpusID:16281709

25. Zhang, Z., Sabuncu, M.R.: Generalized cross entropy loss for training deep neural networks with noisy labels. CoRR **abs/1805.07836** (2018). http://arxiv.org/abs/1805.07836
26. Zhou, T., Canu, S., Vera, P., Ruan, S.: Brain tumor segmentation with missing modalities via latent multi-source correlation representation. In: Medical Image Computing and Computer Assisted Intervention–MICCAI 2020: 23rd International Conference, Lima, Peru, 4–8 October 2020, Proceedings, Part IV 23, pp. 533–541. Springer (2020)

3D MRI Brain Tumor Diagnosis with Topological Descriptors

Hamza Daruger, David J. Brodsky, and Baris Coskunuzer(✉)

University of Texas at Dallas, Richardson, TX 75080, USA
{hamza.daruger,david.brodsky,coskunuz}@utdallas.edu

Abstract. In this paper, we introduce a novel approach that utilizes topological data analysis (TDA) in conjunction with MRI for determining glioma grade and identifying genomic biomarkers. The study hypothesizes that by examining the evolution of topological patterns across various grayscale values, it is possible to identify distinct topological footprints left by different tumor classes in MR images. These footprints can be used as powerful feature vectors for tumor classification. The results of the study demonstrate that higher dimensional topological features provide a powerful ML model, achieving toe-to-toe results with the existing state-of-the-art models in accurately classifying both low- and high-grade gliomas. Additionally, the proposed method achieves high accuracy in predicting the methylation status of the MGMT promoter, which is crucial for prognostic assessment and treatment response prediction. By incorporating TDA output, this research has the potential to advance MRI-based deep learning approaches, enabling the identification of clinically significant tumor features and facilitating informed clinical decision-making.

Keywords: Brain tumor detection · glioma · glioblastoma · MGMT promoter · topological data analysis · cubical persistence · machine learning

1 Introduction

Around 700,000 individuals in the United States are estimated to be living with a primary brain tumor, and it is projected that approximately 90,000 people will receive a primary brain tumor diagnosis in 2022 [45]. Among adults, gliomas are the most common type of primary malignant brain tumors, while in children, they are the leading cause of cancer-related deaths [48]. Upon clinical presentation, patients typically undergo imaging followed by biopsy alone or

H. Daruger and D. J. Brodsky—Equal Contribution.

Supplementary Information The online version contains supplementary material available at https://doi.org/10.1007/978-3-031-76160-7_8.

U. Baid et al. (Eds.): BrainLes 2023/SWITCH 2023, LNCS 14668, pp. 81–94, 2024.
https://doi.org/10.1007/978-3-031-76160-7_8

biopsy with resection for diagnosis and determination of histopathologic classification, tumor grade, and molecular markers [63]. Distinguishing between low-grade gliomas (LGGs; grade II) and high-grade gliomas (HGGs; grades III, IV) is crucial because the prognosis and treatment strategies can vary significantly based on the grade [22,38]. While tissue biopsy is considered the gold standard for diagnosis, it is an invasive procedure that carries risks and can sometimes yield inconclusive results. According to the Cancer Genome Atlas (TCGA) report, only 35% of the biopsy samples contain sufficient tumor content for accurate molecular characterization (Cancer Genome Atlas Research Network, 2008). Therefore, there is a need for reliable non-invasive approaches that can provide accurate diagnosis and monitor tumor progression.

In the past decade, significant progress has been made in machine learning methods, enabling the segmentation of brain tumors and the prediction of their genetic and molecular characteristics based on MRI data [54]. However, despite these advancements, none of the computer vision and machine learning approaches attempted so far have achieved clinical viability due to their limited performance [12]. In order for these models to be useful in clinical settings, usability aspects, including confidence in the output, are of utmost importance [36].

Despite the availability of a large amount of multiparametric data in the BraTS 2021 challenge (n=585), none of the participants, including the top-performing team with a ROC-AUC of 0.62, were able to identify reliable MR imaging features that correlate with MGMT methylation in gliomas [8]. However, a recent study utilized principal component analysis (PCA) on the final convolutional neural network (CNN) layer to extract key imaging features essential for the successful detection of MGMT methylation. The study identified several predictive features, including mixed nodular enhancement, the presence of an eccentric cyst or area of necrosis, mass-like edema with cortical involvement, and slight frontal and superficial temporal predominance [17]. Contrary to these findings, MGMT methylation status in IDH-wild type Glioblastoma was not found to be associated with histopathological or immunohistochemical features such as the degree of proliferation and angiogenesis [43]. Current methods have limitations in effectively utilizing the variability in tumor shape and texture that characterize different types of diffuse gliomas. To address this, the proposal suggests using topological features computed by persistent homology to predict tumor aggressiveness and genetic characteristics. We hypothesize that topological features contain valuable complementary information to image-based features, which can enhance the discriminatory performance of classifiers.

Our contributions.

- We present a fresh perspective on MRI screening for brain tumors by introducing the latest topological data analysis (TDA) approaches to the domain.
- Through the study of higher dimensional topological patterns, we discover that each tumor type exhibits a distinct topological signature in 3D MRI images, enabling the differentiation of various tumor types and grades as well as detecting the presence of MGMT promoter methylation.

- Our model achieves competitive results when compared to the state-of-the-art DL models on benchmark datasets (BRATS 2019 and 2021) on tumor grading and detecting the presence of MGMT promoter methylation.
- Our approach provides an effective feature extraction method and our topological features can easily be integrated with upcoming ML and DL methods in the domain.
- Our proposed topological feature vectors are both explainable and interpretable (Fig. 2 and 3). This provides a viable foundation for new approaches in the early screening of brain tumors (Sect. 4.4).

2 Related Work

2.1 Machine Learning in Brain Tumor Detection

Brain tumor detection plays a crucial role in early diagnosis and treatment planning for patients. Traditional methods of brain tumor detection heavily rely on the expertise of radiologists, leading to variations in accuracy and efficiency. However, with the advent of machine learning techniques, the field of brain tumor detection has witnessed significant advancements. One of the fundamental tasks in brain tumor detection is accurately segmenting the tumor region from the surrounding healthy tissue. Machine learning algorithms, such as convolutional neural networks (CNNs), have demonstrated exceptional performance in automated image segmentation. These algorithms can learn spatial patterns and identify tumor boundaries, facilitating precise tumor localization and measurement. The surveys [39,58] give a nice overview of the state-of-the-art on brain tumor segmentation models. Another important task in brain tumor detection is brain tumor classification. In the past decade, CNN models proved to be quite successful in this aim by learning complex patterns and relationships from the training data, enabling accurate classification of brain tumors based on their characteristics, such as size, shape, and tissue composition. For thorough surveys on recent ML and DL approaches to brain tumor grading and detection, see [6,31,44,60].

On the other hand, RSNA-MICCAI 2021 challenge [8] brought attention to the detection of MGMT promoter methylation problem, where several latest ML models applied in the challenge. Even though it is a binary task, the highest accuracy score was 62% [1]. Some of the works suggested that current DL models fail to obtain a good result on this specific task by trying various CNN models [37, 52]. Other feature extraction methods also fail to give satisfying results on the problem [47]. In this work, we show that topological feature extraction methods outperforms all the existing models.

2.2 TDA in Image Processing

Persistent homology, the main tool in TDA, has been quite effective for pattern recognition in image and shape analysis. There have been several works in various fields in the past two decades, e.g., analysis of images of hepatic lesions [3], human and monkey fibrin images [13], tumor classification [23,46,50], fingerprint classification [29], retinal image analysis [26,28], analysis of 3D shapes [57], neuronal morphology [35], brain angiography [11], fMRI analysis [51,59], genomic data [15]. See also the excellent surveys [55,56] for a thorough review of TDA methods in biomedicine and medical imaging. Note that TDA Applications Library [30] presents hundreds of interesting applications of TDA in various fields.

3 Methodology

3.1 Persistent Homology

TDA has become increasingly popular in a broad range of machine learning tasks, ranging from graph representation learning and manifold learning to image analysis [18]. *Persistent Homology* (PH) being the key approach in TDA provides a unique topological fingerprint of the data by assessing the evolution of various hidden patterns in the data as we vary a scale parameter [62]. While PH can be applied to various forms of data (point clouds, graphs) [25], here we focus only on its use in image settings. This special case is also called *cubical persistence.*

PH process can be described in 3-steps. We consider a 3D MRI image $\mathcal{X}$ (say $r \times s \times t$ resolution), as a 3D cubical complex of size $r \times s \times t$. The first step in PH is to induce a nested sequence of 3D binary images (3D cubical complex). Then, PH keeps track of the topological features (connected components, holes/loops, and cavities) in this sequence of binary images [21,34]. To create such sequence, one can use grayscale values $\gamma_{ijk} \in [0, 255]$ of each voxel $\Delta_{ijk} \subset \mathcal{X}$. Then, for a sequence of grayscale values ($0 \leq t_1 < t_2 < \cdots < t_N \leq 255$), one obtains 3D binary images $\mathcal{X}_1 \subset \mathcal{X}_2 \subset \cdots \subset \mathcal{X}_N$ where $\mathcal{X}_n = \{\Delta_{ijk} \subset \mathcal{X} \mid \gamma_{ijk} \leq t_n\}$. In other words, we start with an empty (all-white) 3D image of size $r \times s \times t$ and keep activating (coloring black) the voxels when their grayscale value passes the given threshold at each step. This is called *sublevel filtration* for $\mathcal{X}$ with respect to a given function (grayscale in this case).

In the second step, PH keeps track of the evolution of topological features in this sequence of cubical complexes $\{\mathcal{X}_n\}$, and records it as *persistence diagram* (PD). In particular, if a topological feature σ first appears in $\mathcal{X}_m$ and disappears in $\mathcal{X}_n$, we call $b_\sigma = t_m$ *birth time* and $d_\sigma = t_n$ *the death*

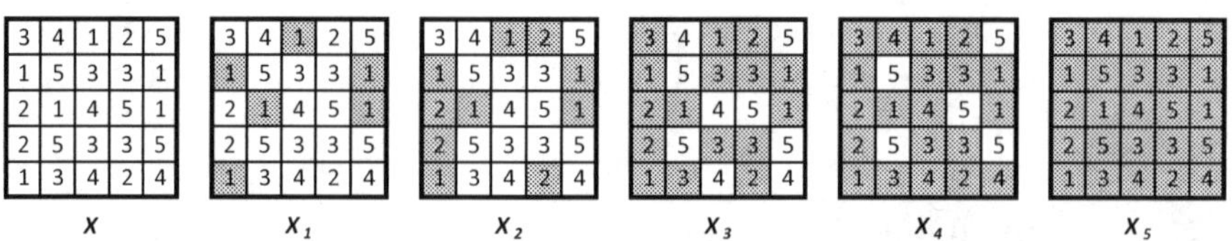

Fig. 1. Sublevel filtration. The leftmost figure represents an image of 5×5 size with the given pixel values. Then, the sublevel filtration is the sequence of binary images $\mathcal{X}_1 \subset \mathcal{X}_2 \subset \mathcal{X}_3 \subset \mathcal{X}_4 \subset \mathcal{X}_5$.

time of the topological feature σ. Then, PD is the collection of all such 2-tuples $\mathrm{PD}_k(\mathcal{X}) = \{(b_\sigma, d_\sigma)\}$ where k represent the dimension of the topological features. e.g., in Fig. 1, for dimension-0 (connected components), we have $\mathrm{PD}_0(\mathcal{X}) = \{(1,\infty),(1,3),(1,2),(1,2),(2,3)\}$ while dimension-1 (holes), we have $\mathrm{PD}_1(\mathcal{X}) = \{(3,5),(3,5),(4,5)\}$. As $\mathcal{X}$ is 2D, $\mathrm{PD}_2(\mathcal{X}) = \emptyset$.

In real-life applications, working directly with persistence diagrams (PDs) as collections of 2-tuples can be challenging when integrating with ML tools. Therefore, a common approach is to convert the PD information into a vector or a function, a process known as *vectorization* [4], which serves as the final step of the persistent homology (PH) process. One commonly used function for vectorization is the *Betti function*, which effectively tracks the number of "alive" topological features at a given threshold. Specifically, the Betti function is a step function where $\beta_0(t_n)$ represents the count of connected components in the binary image $\mathcal{X}_n$, $\beta_1(t_n)$ denotes the number of holes (loops) in $\mathcal{X}_n$, and $\beta_2(t_n)$ representing the count of voids in $\mathcal{X}_n$. In ML applications, Betti functions are often represented as vectors $\boldsymbol{\beta}_k$ of size N with entries $\beta_k(t_n)$ for $1 \leq n \leq N$. Thus, we have $\boldsymbol{\beta}_k(\mathcal{X}) = [\beta_k(t_1)\ \beta_k(t_2)\ \ldots\ \beta_k(t_N)]$.

For example, considering 2D toy example $\mathcal{X}$ in Fig. 1, we obtain $\boldsymbol{\beta}_0(\mathcal{X}) = [4\ 3\ 1\ 1\ 1]$ and $\boldsymbol{\beta}_1(\mathcal{X}) = [0\ 0\ 2\ 3\ 0]$. Here, $\beta_0(1) = 4$ represents the count of components in $\mathcal{X}_1$, while $\beta_1(3) = 2$ denotes the count of holes (loops) in $\mathcal{X}_3$. Since the image is 2D, $\boldsymbol{\beta}_2(\mathcal{X})$ is trivial, however in 3D images, $\boldsymbol{\beta}_2(\mathcal{X})$ captures the key features as it counts the voids in binary images $\{\mathcal{X}_n\}$. It is worth noting that there exist other methods to convert PDs into vectors, such as Persistence Images [2], Persistence Landscapes [14], and Silhouettes [19]. However, in order to maintain interpretability in our model, we deliberately chose to employ Betti functions in this work (see Sect. 4.4).

3.2 Topological Footprints of Tumors in MRI

To extract the topological features, for a given 3D MRI image $\mathcal{X}$ (say $r \times s \times t$ size), we first extract all grayscale values for 4 modalities of 3D MRI images for $\mathcal{X}$, i.e., T1, T2, T1-weighted, and Flair. In other words, we produce four grayscale functions $\mathbf{T}_1(i,j,k)$, $\mathbf{T}_2(i,j,k)$, $\mathbf{T}_{1w}(i,j,k)$, $\mathbf{F}(i,j,k)$ where each function $f(i,j,k)$ assigns every voxel $\Delta_{ijk} \subset \mathcal{X}$ to its assigned grayscale value for $1 \leq i \leq r$, $1 \leq j \leq s$ and $1 \leq k \leq t$.

After defining these four functions corresponding to MRI modalities, we construct a sublevel filtration for each grayscale function $f(i,j,k)$, and obtain the corresponding persistence diagrams $\mathrm{PD}_k(\mathcal{X}, f)$ for dimensions $k = 0, 1, 2$ as explained in Sect. 3.1. In our experiments, we choose the number of thresholds as $N = 100$, i.e., $t_1 = 0$ and $t_{100} = 255$ with $t_n = (\frac{255}{99}).(n-1)$. In a way, we renormalized the grayscale range $[0, 255]$ into $[1, 100]$. Therefore, we get a filtration of length 100, i.e. $\mathcal{X}_1^f \subset \mathcal{X}_2^f \subset \cdots \subset \mathcal{X}_{100}^f$ where $\mathcal{X}_n^f$ is the 3D binary image where the voxels Δ_{ijk} with grayscale value $f(i,j,k) \leq t_n$. Then, for each MRI modality (T1, T2, T1-weighted, and Flair), we obtain our three feature vectors $\boldsymbol{\beta}_0^f, \boldsymbol{\beta}_1^f, \boldsymbol{\beta}_2^f$ where each one of them is 100 dimensional (See Fig. 1). In particular, $\beta_0^f(t_n)$ is the count of distinct components in binary 3D image $\mathcal{X}_n^f$, $\beta_1(t_n)$ is the count of distinct holes (loops) in $\mathcal{X}_n^f$ and finally $\beta_2^f(t_n)$ is the count of cavities in $\mathcal{X}_n^f$. For example, if $f = \mathbf{T}_2$, $\beta_1^{T_2}(t_n)$ represents number of *loops* in 3D binary image $\mathcal{X}_n^{T_2}$. Similarly, for $f = \mathbf{F}$, $\beta_2^F(t_n)$ represents number of *cavities* in 3D binary image $\mathcal{X}_n^F$. Hence, three 100-dimensional vectors for four MRI modalities provide 1200 features for each patient. By choosing the number of thresholds (N) differently, one can obtain different-size feature vectors. Note that it is possible to choose thresholds in a non-linear way. One fine way to do it is to analyze the outcome of initial thresholding and restrict the new thresholds in a smaller interval of interest with finer resolution.

From ML perspective, our feature extraction method can be considered as an image embedding technique. For each MRI image, we obtain 100-dimensional Betti-0, 100-dimensional Betti-1 and 100-dimensional Betti-12 vectors. These vectors allow us to embed each image into the latent space $\mathbb{R}^{100}$ (or $\mathbb{R}^{300}$ when all vectors are used). The width of the confidence bands indicates that each class tends to aggregate in a single cluster within the latent space for these feature vectors. Typically, in classification problems of this nature, different ML methods attempt to distinguish various clusters that form within each class using diverse algorithms. In our particular case, one can perceive the median curves as the center of each cluster representing a class, and the feature vectors of the images within that class are positioned close by in the latent (feature) space.

3.3 ML Model

We give the specific details of our ML Model in Sect. 4. In particular, we used one of the open-source auto-ML models, Pycaret, which covers various ML models, including tree-based models, SVM, KNN, GDA, Logistic regression and many others. We also used feature selection and feed-forward neural network (MLP) models to apply to our topological features.

4 Experiments

4.1 Datasets

BraTS 2019 dataset[1] consists of 335 3D brain MRI scans, segmented manually by one to four experienced neuroradiologists ensuring consistency in the tumor annotation protocol [9,10,40,42]. 259 of them belong to patients diagnosed with HGG and 76 of them to those diagnosed with LGG. Segmentation annotations comprise four classes: the necrotic and non-enhancing tumor core (NCR/NET–label 1), the peritumoral edema (ED–label 2), background (voxels that are not part of the tumor–label 3) and GD-enhancing tumor (ET–label 4). Each MRI scan image has 4 modalities: native (T1) and post-contrast T1-weighted (T1Gd), T2-weighted (T2), and d) T2 Fluid Attenuated Inversion Recovery (FLAIR) and

[1] https://www.med.upenn.edu/cbica/brats2019/data.html.

each modality has dimensions of (240, 240, 155) voxels. The provided data is skull-stripped and interpolated to the same resolution of 1 mm^3.

BraTS 2021 Benchmark Dataset on Radiogenomic Classification is coming from a public challenge[2] that consists of 585 3D brain MRI scans comprised of modalities: T1, T1Gd, T2 and T2-FLAIR with xy-dimensions of (512, 512) voxels [8] and varying sizes of z-dimension (depth) across different scand id's and modalities. Similar to BRATS 2019 dataset, preprocessing includes coregistration of the images to the same anatomical template, resampling to a uniform isotroping resolution of 1 mm^3 and skull-stripping. Each MRI scan is associated with the MGMT promoter methylation status, which is defined as a binary label (0: unmethylated, 1: methylated). It is a balanced dataset with 278 unmethylated with 307 methylated labels.

4.2 Experimental Setup

All the current state-of-the-art models on these datasets mostly use CNNs whereas our studies are based on standard ML models that can be trained much faster than DL models. In both the BraTS 2019 and BraTS 2021 datasets, for each MRI, we used Giotto-TDA [61] to generate $\mathrm{PD}_k(\mathcal{X}, f)$ for dimensions $k = 0, 1, 2$ for each of the 4 MRI modalities, as explained above. After randomly splitting the dataset using a $80 : 20$ train-test split, we generated feature vectors using two versions of thresholding. In the first, the thresholds are scaled to each MRI, i.e., t_1 and t_{100} are the earliest birth times and latest death times for that particular MRI. In the other, thresholds are scaled to the entire training dataset, i.e., t_1 and t_{100} are the earliest birth times and latest death times for all MRIs with that channel.

After obtaining the 1200 dimensional feature vectors for each MRI, we used PyCaret's AutoML tools [5] to perform feature selection and create simple ML models. We provided the performance of our model with other ML classifiers in Pycaret in Tables 3 and 4 in Supplementary Material. Alongside the Betti functions we computed the power-weighted Silhouettes of $\mathrm{PD}_k(\mathcal{X}, f)$ using powers $\frac{1}{2}$, 1, 2 as an alternative vectorization. Note that we used the whole MRI images, and no segmentation maps are used when obtaining our vectorizations. Additionally, along with the simple ML models, we trained a 3-layer MLP using the Scikit-learn library [49]. For both datasets, we obtained our best results with Betti vectorizations and tree-based models in Pycaret AutoML tools (Adaboost for BRATS 2019, and Random Forest for BRATS 2021). We provided more details on our models and their performances in Supp. Material.

The computation to generate persistence diagrams, the vectorization, and the training of the ML models were done on a system with an Intel Core i7-12700k and 32 GB Memory. The time to process the 335 images of the BraTS 2019 dataset into the Betti vectors was 4.5 h. We provide our code in the link at the link[3].

---

2 https://www.kaggle.com/c/rsna-miccai-brain-tumor-radiogenomic-classification.

3 https://anonymous.4open.science/r/3D-TDA-MRI-0B46.

4.3 Results

In Tables 1 and 2, we report our accuracy results for our Topological ML model along with the latest models on the problems. We directly used the reported accuracy values in the given references for each model. In Table 1, all the models use the same dataset (BRATS 2019) with 335 (259:76) MRI images. In Table 2, all models use the same dataset BRATS 2021 except the first two models [37] (combining another dataset with BRATS 2021). Note that deep learning models use various data augmentation methods. As our topological feature vectors are invariant under rotation, translation, and flipping, we did not use any data augmentation methods in this study.

In Table 1, our topological ML model gives competitive results in HGG vs. LGG detection with the latest deep learning models. Considering that this is an unbalanced dataset, being in the top three AUC scores shows the good performance of the model.

On the other hand, in Table 2, we observe that our topological feature vectors outperform all SOTA models by a significant margin. Note that in BRATS 2021 challenge, the highest accuracy result was 62% [1]. In the next couple of years, several deep learning models are applied to this difficult problem, but they all fail to pass the 70% threshold in accuracy. These results indicate that higher dimensional topological patterns can be quite useful in brain tumor grading and detection.

4.4 Explainability and Interpretability

Gliomas present a diverse range of characteristics on conventional imaging, which are influenced by factors like tumor grade, location, and molecular subtypes. Glioblastomas (Grade IV tumors) are commonly identified by their irregular margins, intricate enhancement patterns, and the presence of necrosis, edema, and varying degrees of intratumoral hemorrhage. These features can be effectively captured using a combination of T2-weighted and gadolinium

Table 1. Accuracy results for Glioma grading on BraTS 2019 dataset.

BraTS 2019 Dataset					
Method	**Train:Test**	**Prec**	**Recall**	**Acc**	**AUC**
AlexNet [33]	80:20	–	–	–	0.83
Wavelets [41]	80:20	**90.4**	73.0	<u>90.7</u>	0.85
L-UNet [64]	80:20	–	89.5	89.3	0.89
ResNet18 [32]	85:15	–	<u>94.9</u>	90.5	0.92
SqNet [32]	85:15	–	94.0	89.0	0.90
D-CNN [32]	85:15	–	**98.4**	**96.9**	<u>0.97</u>
GAP [65]	80:20	–	–	–	**0.98**
Topo-ML	80:20	<u>89.1</u>	94.2	86.6	0.92

Table 2. Accuracy results for MGMT promoter detection on BraTS 2021 dataset.

BraTS 2019 Dataset					
Method	**Train:Test**	**Prec**	**Recall**	**Acc**	**AUC**
AlexNet [33]	80:20	–	–	–	0.83
Wavelets [41]	80:20	**90.4**	73.0	<u>90.7</u>	0.85
L-UNet [64]	80:20	–	89.5	89.3	0.89
ResNet18 [32]	85:15	–	<u>94.9</u>	90.5	0.92
SqNet [32]	85:15	–	94.0	89.0	0.90
D-CNN [32]	85:15	–	**98.4**	**96.9**	<u>0.97</u>
GAP [65]	80:20	–	–	–	**0.98**
Topo-ML	80:20	<u>89.1</u>	94.2	86.6	0.92

contrast-enhanced T1-weighted MRI sequences. Additionally, MRI can detect other aspects such as subependymal or leptomeningeal spread of the tumor, as well as diffuse infiltration involving multiple brain locations.

In contrast, LGGs like astrocytomas and oligodendrogliomas are often non-enhancing and have well-defined boundaries. However, anaplastic astrocytomas and oligodendrogliomas may exhibit overlapping imaging findings with both LGG and glioblastoma. Although anatomic MRI is quite sensitive in detecting brain lesions, it lacks specificity for tumors, and heterogeneity exists within and among grades. Notably, a significant percentage of supratentorial gliomas (14–45%) that do not show enhancement on post-gadolinium T1-weighted images are malignant, and up to 25% of high-grade gliomas display only faint or no detectable enhancement [7,53].

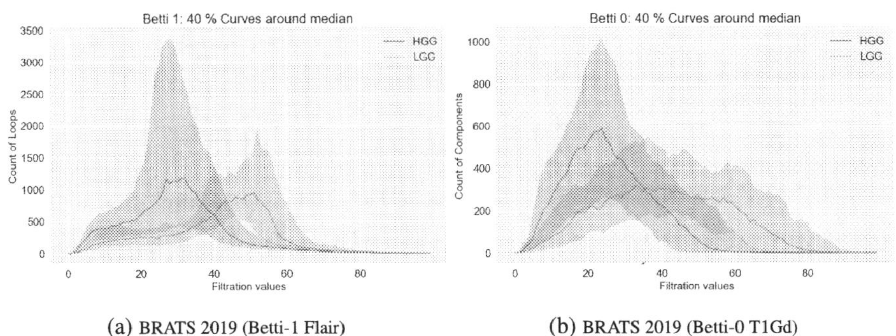

(a) BRATS 2019 (Betti-1 Flair)

(b) BRATS 2019 (Betti-0 T1Gd)

Fig. 2. Glioma. Median curves and 40% confidence bands of our topological feature vectors (Betti functions) for BRATS 2019 for Glioma diagnosis. x-axis represents grayscale values and y-axis represents count of components (Betti-0), count of loops (Betti-1) or count of voids (Betti-2) in the corresponding binary images. See Sect. 4.4 for details and interpretation.

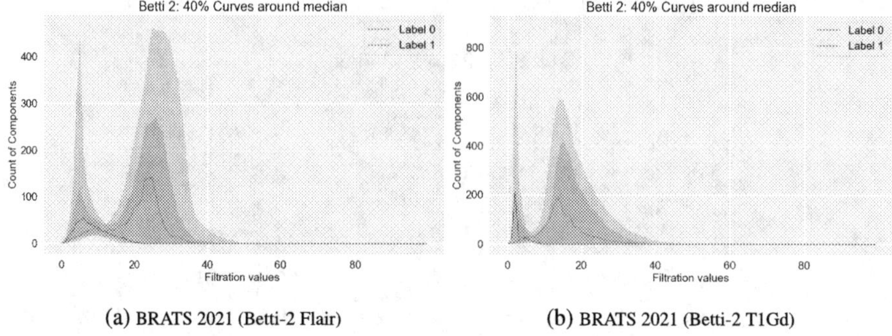

(a) BRATS 2021 (Betti-2 Flair)

(b) BRATS 2021 (Betti-2 T1Gd)

Fig. 3. MGMT. Median curves and 40% confidence bands of our topological feature vectors (Betti functions) for BRATS 2021 for MGMT detection. x-axis represents grayscale values and y-axis represents count of components (Betti-0), count of loops (Betti-1) or count of voids (Betti-2) in the corresponding binary images. See Sect. 4.4 for details and interpretation.

Topological features offer a promising approach to highlight regions with significant biological properties, such as increased cellularity, microvascular hyperplasia, proliferation, and hypoxia, which conventional imaging approaches might miss. 3D arrays of gray-scale values in the tumor can reveal distinct geometric patterns associated with specific tumor characteristics. These patterns can be captured by TPA (Tumor Pattern Analysis), potentially aiding in the differential diagnosis of gliomas.

Figures 2 and 3 depict the different topological features induced by normal and abnormal classes in the corresponding datasets. Recall that Betti-0 represents the number of connected components. In particular, in Fig. 2b, we observe that while HGG class develops almost 600 components in the binary images for T1Gd MRI with threshold 20 (grayscale $\sim$50), LGG class barely develops about one-third of it, about 200 components. On the other hand in lighter regions, while HGG class becomes almost completely connected (the number of components is only a few) around threshold 60 (grayscale $\sim$150), LGG class is still highly disconnected with about 200 components. Similarly, in Fig. 3a, we observe that the number of cavities (Betti-2) for the methylated class are much larger than the unmethylated class in the binary images from Flair MRI with threshold 20 (grayscale $\sim$50).

4.5 Limitations

While the method gives outstanding performance compared to the state-of-the-art models in MGMT promoter detection, it falls behind in tumor grading. One of the main reasons is that topological feature extraction methods are agnostic to standard data augmentation methods, and one needs to use minority oversampling methods carefully to improve the model performance.

5 Discussion

In this study, we have successfully integrated topological data analysis tools into the analysis of brain tumors. Our novel method for extracting topological features from 3D MRI images has shown great promise in accurately grading tumors and detecting MGMT promoters. The information provided by these topological patterns complements existing methods, suggesting that integrating topological feature vectors into CNN models could significantly enhance their performance. Moving forward, our future projects will center on further exploring this direction to create a robust clinical decision support system in this domain. By leveraging the power of topological data analysis alongside the latest deep learning techniques, we aim to develop an effective and reliable clinical decision support system for brain tumor analysis.

Acknowledgements. This work was supported by grants from the National Science Foundation (Grants # DMS-2202584, DMS-2220613, DMS-2229417), and from the Simons Foundation (Grant # 579977).

References

1. BRATS 2021 challenge. https://www.kaggle.com/competitions/rsna-miccai-brain-tumor-radiogenomic-classification/
2. Adams, H., et al.: Persistence images: a stable vector representation of persistent homology. J. Mach. Learn. Res. **18**(1), 218–252 (2017)
3. Adcock, A., Rubin, D., Carlsson, G.: Classification of hepatic lesions using the matching metric. Comput. Vis. Image Underst. **121**, 36–42 (2014)
4. Ali, D., et al.: A survey of vectorization methods in topological data analysis. arXiv preprint arXiv:2212.09703 (2022)
5. Ali, M.: PyCaret: an open source, low-code machine learning library in Python, April 2020. https://www.pycaret.org, pyCaret version 1.0.0
6. Amin, J., Sharif, M., Haldorai, A., Yasmin, M., Nayak, R.S.: Brain tumor detection and classification using machine learning: a comprehensive survey. Complex Intell. Syst. 1–23 (2021)
7. Baehring, J.M., Bi, W.L., Bannykh, S., Piepmeier, J.M., Fulbright, R.K.: Diffusion mri in the early diagnosis of malignant glioma. J. Neurooncol. **82**, 221–225 (2007)
8. Baid, U., et al.: The RSNA-ASNR-MICCAI BRATS 2021 benchmark on brain tumor segmentation and radiogenomic classification. arXiv preprint arXiv:2107.02314 (2021)
9. Bakas, S., et al.: Segmentation labels for the pre-operative scans of the tcga-gbm collection. The cancer imaging archive (2017)
10. Bakas, S., et al.: Identifying the best machine learning algorithms for brain tumor segmentation, progression assessment, and overall survival prediction in the BRATS challenge. arXiv preprint arXiv:1811.02629 (2018)
11. Bendich, P., Marron, J.S., Miller, E., Pieloch, A., Skwerer, S.: Persistent homology analysis of brain artery trees. Ann. Appl. Stat. **10**(1), 198 (2016)
12. Benjamens, S., Dhunnoo, P., Meskó, B.: The state of artificial intelligence-based FDA-approved medical devices and algorithms: an online database. NPJ Digit. Med. **3**(1), 1–8 (2020)

13. Berry, E., Chen, Y.C., Cisewski-Kehe, J., Fasy, B.T.: Functional summaries of persistence diagrams. J. Appl. Comput. Topol. **4**(2), 211–262 (2020)
14. Bubenik, P., et al.: Statistical topological data analysis using persistence landscapes. J. Mach. Learn. Res. **16**(1), 77–102 (2015)
15. Cámara, P.G., Levine, A.J., Rabadan, R.: Inference of ancestral recombination graphs through topological data analysis. PLoS Comput. Biol. **12**(8), e1005071 (2016)
16. Capuozzo, S., Gravina, M., Gatta, G., Marrone, S., Sansone, C.: A multimodal knowledge-based deep learning approach for mgmt promoter methylation identification. J. Imaging **8**(12), 321 (2022)
17. Chang, P., et al.: Deep-learning convolutional neural networks accurately classify genetic mutations in gliomas. Am. J. Neuroradiol. **39**(7), 1201–1207 (2018)
18. Chazal, F., Michel, B.: An introduction to topological data analysis: fundamental and practical aspects for data scientists. Front. Artif. Intell. **4** (2021)
19. Chazal, F., Fasy, B.T., Lecci, F., Rinaldo, A., Wasserman, L.: Stochastic convergence of persistence landscapes and silhouettes. In: Proceedings of the Thirtieth Annual Symposium on Computational Geometry, pp. 474–483 (2014)
20. Chen, D.T., Chen, A.T., Wang, H.: Simple and fast convolutional neural network applied to median cross sections for predicting the presence of mgmt promoter methylation in flair mri scans. In: International MICCAI Brainlesion Workshop, pp. 227–238. Springer (2021)
21. Choe, S., Ramanna, S.: Cubical homology-based machine learning: an application in image classification. Axioms **11**(3), 112 (2022)
22. Claus, E.B., et al.: Survival and low-grade glioma: the emergence of genetic information. Neurosurg. Focus **38**(1), E6 (2015)
23. Crawford, L., Monod, A., Chen, A.X., Mukherjee, S., Rabadán, R.: Predicting clinical outcomes in glioblastoma: an application of topological and functional data analysis. J. Am. Stat. Assoc. **115**(531), 1139–1150 (2020)
24. Das, S.: Optimizing prediction of mgmt promoter methylation from mri scans using adversarial learning. In: 2022 IEEE 34th International Conference on Tools with Artificial Intelligence (ICTAI), pp. 1047–1054. IEEE (2022)
25. Dey, T.K., Wang, Y.: Computational Topology for Data Analysis. Cambridge University Press (2022)
26. Dunaeva, O., Edelsbrunner, H., Lukyanov, A., Machin, M., Malkova, D., Kuvaev, R., Kashin, S.: The classification of endoscopy images with persistent homology. Pattern Recogn. Lett. **83**, 13–22 (2016)
27. Faghani, S., Khosravi, B., Moassefi, M., Conte, G.M., Erickson, B.J.: A comparison of three different deep learning-based models to predict the mgmt promoter methylation status in glioblastoma using brain mri. Journal of Digital Imaging, pp. 1–10 (2023)
28. Garside, K., Henderson, R., Makarenko, I., Masoller, C.: Topological data analysis of high resolution diabetic retinopathy images. PLoS ONE **14**(5), e0217413 (2019)
29. Giansiracusa, N., Giansiracusa, R., Moon, C.: Persistent homology machine learning for fingerprint classification. In: 2019 18th IEEE International Conference On Machine Learning And Applications (ICMLA), pp. 1219–1226. IEEE (2019)
30. Giunti, B.: Tda applications library (2022). https://www.zotero.org/groups/2425412/tda-applications/library
31. Gull, S., Akbar, S.: Artificial intelligence in brain tumor detection through mri scans: In: Advancements and Challenges. Artificial Intelligence and Internet of Things, pp. 241–276 (2021)

32. Hafeez, H.A., et al.: A CNN-model to classify low-grade and high-grade glioma from mri images. IEEE Access (2023)
33. Hao, R., Namdar, K., Liu, L., Khalvati, F.: A transfer learning-based active learning framework for brain tumor classification. Front. Artif. Intell. **4**, 635766 (2021)
34. Kaji, S., Sudo, T., Ahara, K.: Cubical ripser: software for computing persistent homology of image and volume data. arXiv preprint arXiv:2005.12692 (2020)
35. Kanari, L., et al.: A topological representation of branching neuronal morphologies. Neuroinformatics **16**(1), 3–13 (2018)
36. Kelly, C.J., Karthikesalingam, A., Suleyman, M., Corrado, G., King, D.: Key challenges for delivering clinical impact with artificial intelligence. BMC Med. **17**(1), 1–9 (2019)
37. Kim, B.H., Lee, H., Choi, K.S., Nam, J.G., Park, C.K., Park, S.H., Chung, J.W., Choi, S.H.: Validation of mri-based models to predict mgmt promoter methylation in gliomas: Brats 2021 radiogenomics challenge. Cancers **14**(19), 4827 (2022)
38. Lacroix, M., Abi-Said, D., Fourney, D.R., Gokaslan, Z.L., Shi, W., DeMonte, F., Lang, F.F., McCutcheon, I.E., Hassenbusch, S.J., Holland, E., et al.: A multivariate analysis of 416 patients with glioblastoma multiforme: prognosis, extent of resection, and survival. J. Neurosurg. **95**(2), 190–198 (2001)
39. Liu, Z., et al.: Deep learning based brain tumor segmentation: a survey. Complex Intell. Syst. **9**(1), 1001–1026 (2023)
40. Lloyd, C.T., Sorichetta, A., Tatem, A.J.: High resolution global gridded data for use in population studies. Sci. Data **4**(1), 1–17 (2017)
41. Mathews, C., Mohamed, A.: Deep classification of glioma grade using 3d wavelet features. In: 2022 International Conference for Advancement in Technology (ICONAT), pp. 1–5. IEEE (2022)
42. Menze, J., et al.: A comparison of random forest and its gini importance with standard chemometric methods for the feature selection and classification of spectral data, BMC Bioinf. **10**(1) (2009)
43. Mikkelsen, V.E., et al.: Mgmt promoter methylation status is not related to histological or radiological features in idh wild-type glioblastomas. J. Neuropathol. Exp. Neurol. **79**(8), 855–862 (2020)
44. Muhammad, K., Khan, S., Del Ser, J., De Albuquerque, V.H.C.: Deep learning for multigrade brain tumor classification in smart healthcare systems: a prospective survey. IEEE Trans. Neural Netw. Learn. Syst. **32**(2), 507–522 (2020)
45. Ostrom, Q.T., Cioffi, G., Waite, K., Kruchko, C., Barnholtz-Sloan, J.S.: Cbtrus statistical report: primary brain and other central nervous system tumors diagnosed in the united states in 2014–2018. Neuro-oncology **23**(Supplement_3), iii1–iii105 (2021)
46. Oyama, A., et al.: Hepatic tumor classification using texture and topology analysis of non-contrast-enhanced three-dimensional t1-weighted mr images with a radiomics approach. Sci. Rep. **9**(1), 1–10 (2019)
47. Pálsson, S., Cerri, S., Van Leemput, K.: Prediction of mgmt methylation status of glioblastoma using radiomics and latent space shape features. In: International MICCAI Brainlesion Workshop, pp. 222–231. Springer (2021)
48. Patil, N., et al.: Epidemiology of brainstem high-grade gliomas in children and adolescents in the united states, 2000–2017. Neuro Oncol. **23**(6), 990–998 (2021)
49. Pedregosa, F., et al.: Scikit-learn: machine learning in Python. J. Mach. Learn. Res. **12**, 2825–2830 (2011)
50. Qaiser, T., et al.: Fast and accurate tumor segmentation of histology images using persistent homology and deep convolutional features. Med. Image Anal. **55**, 1–14 (2019)

51. Rieck, B., et al.: Uncovering the topology of time-varying fmri data using cubical persistence. Adv. Neural. Inf. Process. Syst. **33**, 6900–6912 (2020)
52. Saeed, N., Hardan, S., Abutalip, K., Yaqub, M.: Is it possible to predict mgmt promoter methylation from brain tumor mri scans using deep learning models? In: International Conference on Medical Imaging with Deep Learning, pp. 1005–1018. PMLR (2022)
53. Scott, J., Brasher, P., Sevick, R., Rewcastle, N., Forsyth, P.: How often are nonenhancing supratentorial gliomas malignant? a population study. Neurology **59**(6), 947–949 (2002)
54. Shaver, M.M., et al.: Optimizing neuro-oncology imaging: a review of deep learning approaches for glioma imaging. Cancers **11**(6), 829 (2019)
55. Singh, Y., et al.: Topological data analysis in medical imaging: current state of the art. Insights Imaging **14**(1), 1–10 (2023)
56. Skaf, Y., Laubenbacher, R.: Topological data analysis in biomedicine: a review. J. Biomed. Inf. 104082 (2022)
57. Skraba, P., Ovsjanikov, M., Chazal, F., Guibas, L.: Persistence-based segmentation of deformable shapes. In: 2010 IEEE Computer Society Conference on Computer Vision and Pattern Recognition-Workshops, pp. 45–52. IEEE (2010)
58. Soomro, T.A., Zheng, L., Afifi, A.J., Ali, A., Soomro, S., Yin, M., Gao, J.: Image segmentation for mr brain tumor detection using machine learning: a review. IEEE Rev. Biomed. Eng. (2022)
59. Stolz, B.J., Emerson, T., Nahkuri, S., Porter, M.A., Harrington, H.A.: Topological data analysis of task-based fmri data from experiments on schizophrenia. J. Phys. Complexity **2**(3), 035006 (2021)
60. Taha, A.M., Ariffin, D., Abu-Naser, S.S.: A systematic literature review of deep and machine learning algorithms in brain tumor and meta-analysis. J. Theor. Appl. Inf. Technol. **101**(1), 21–36 (2023)
61. Tauzin, G., et al.: giotto-tda: a topological data analysis toolkit for machine learning and data exploration (2020)
62. Wasserman, L.: Topological data analysis. Ann. Rev. Stat. Appl. **5**, 501–532 (2018)
63. Weller, M., et al.: Eano guidelines on the diagnosis and treatment of diffuse gliomas of adulthood. Nat. Rev. Clin. Oncol. **18**(3), 170–186 (2021)
64. Yu, X., et al.: A lightweight 3d unet model for glioma grading. Phys. Med. Biol. **67**(15), 155006 (2022)
65. Zhu, J., Wang, S., He, J., Schönlieb, C.B., Yu, L.: Multi-task learning-driven volume and slice level contrastive learning for 3d medical image classification. In: International Workshop on Computational Mathematics Modeling in Cancer Analysis, pp. 110–120. Springer (2022)

SWITCH

An Automatic Cascaded Model for Hemorrhagic Stroke Segmentation and Hemorrhagic Volume Estimation

Weijin Xu[1], Zhuang Sha[2], Huihua Yang[1(✉)], Rongcai Jiang[2], Zhanying Li[3], Wentao Liu[1], and Ruisheng Su[4]

[1] Beijing University of Posts and Telecommunications, Beijing, China
{xwj1994,yhh}@bupt.edu.cn

[2] Department of Neurosurgery, Tianjin Medical University General Hospital, Tianjin, China

[3] Department of Neurosurgery, Kailuan General Hospital, Tangshan, China

[4] Erasmus MC, Rotterdam, Netherlands

Abstract. Hemorrhagic Stroke (HS) has a rapid onset and is a serious condition that poses a great health threat. Promptly and accurately delineating the bleeding region and estimating the volume of bleeding in Computer Tomography (CT) images can assist clinicians in treatment planning, leading to improved treatment outcomes for patients. In this paper, a cascaded 3D model is constructed based on UNet to perform a two-stage segmentation of the hemorrhage area in CT images from rough to fine, and the hemorrhage volume is automatically calculated from the segmented area. On a dataset with 341 cases of hemorrhagic stroke CT scans, the proposed model provides high-quality segmentation outcome with higher accuracy (DSC 85.66%) and better computation efficiency (6.2 s per sample) when compared to the traditional Tada formula with respect to hemorrhage volume estimation.

Keywords: Hemorrhagic stroke · CT · Hemorrhagic volume estimation · Deep learning · Medical image segmentation

1 Introduction

Stroke is the world's number one deadly and second most disabling disease, posing a huge threat to people's health and a huge burden to the healthcare system [1]. Stroke can be divided into Ischemic Stroke (IS) and Hemorrhagic Stroke (HS), with a high incidence (about 70%) of IS and a relatively low incidence (about 30%) of HS. However, HS is characterized by its rapid onset, grave nature, and significantly higher mortality rate. HS refers to cerebral hemorrhage caused by non-traumatic rupture of blood vessels in the brain parenchyma, and

W. Xu and Z. Sha—Contribute equally.

H. Yang and R. Jiang—are co corresponding authors.

U. Baid et al. (Eds.): BrainLes 2023/SWITCH 2023, LNCS 14668, pp. 97–105, 2024.
https://doi.org/10.1007/978-3-031-76160-7_9

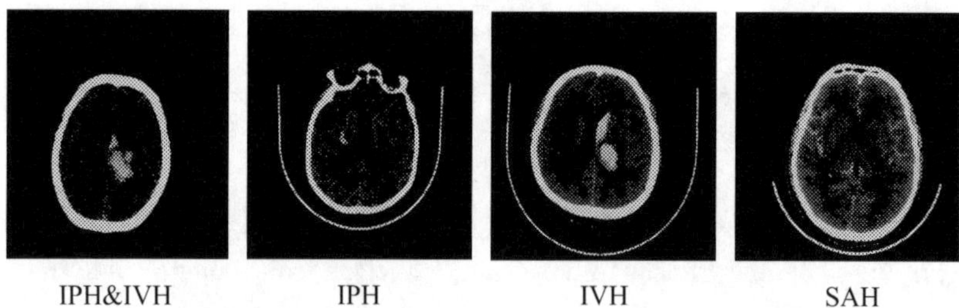

Fig. 1. Sample displays of different types of bleeding, with red masks indicating the bleeding area, where IPH & IVH means the hybrid hemorrhage type of IPH and IVH. Best view in color. (Color figure online)

it contains three types of brain hemorrhage: subarachnoid hemorrhage (SAH), intraparenchymal hemorrhage (IPH), and intraventricular hemorrhage (IVH), as shown in Fig. 1.

The most common causes are hypertension, cerebral atherosclerosis, intracranial vascular malformations, which are often triggered by exertion and emotional excitement [2]. The prime treatment time for the onset of hemorrhagic stroke is within 3 h after the onset. Therefore, timely and rapid determination of the amount, site, and contour of bleeding can bring better treatment results, fewer complications, and less severe sequelae to the patient [4].

The choice of diagnostic methods in each specific case strongly depends not only on their applicability (availability, contraindications, patient's condition, etc.), but also on the time of symptom onset. Any delay in medical care increases the risk of severe consequences and death [7]. Computer Tomography (CT) is used as a first-line diagnostic modality because of its short imaging time, ease of acquisition, high sensitivity to bleeding, high resolution, and clear anatomic relationships. The physicians need to inspect the CT scan and make the appropriate treatment plan depending on the type of bleeding, the area of bleeding, and the size of the bleeding, which takes effort and may present human error in identifying hemorrhages. Therefore, this paper constructs an automated pipeline based on convolutional neural networks (CNNs) to outline the bleeding area in CT, which may reduce the workload of physicians, speed up the diagnosis process, and bring better treatment for patients.

2 Related Work

In [10], a novel artifcial neural network framework method is proposed for detecting the presence or absence of intracranial hemorrhage (ICH) and classifying the type of hemorrhage on CT images of the brain, achieving a performance of AUC 0.859 for detection and AUC 0.903 for classification among 250 CT images (100 healthy, 150 hemorrhage), respectively. RADnet [6] utilizes a 2D CNN to extract the information from the frame-by-frame CT images, then uses Bil-LSTM to fuse the inter-frame dimension-only information, and finally determines whether there is a cerebral hemorrhage in the input CT sequence. In [11], a publicly available 2D dataset of CT frames (752,803 dcms), RSNA, for hemorrhage type classification, RSNA, was proposed, and a baseline ResNet-based classification method was constructed, which ultimately achieved a 93% multi-category classification accuracy. IHA-Net [13] proposed a residual hybrid atrous module to capture features for multiple receptive fields of different sizes and utilizes the idea of deep supervision to add constraints to the middle layer of the network, which makes the network converge faster. HMOE-Net [7] proposed a shallow-deep feature extraction network to deal with hybrid multi-scale object features. Although these methods have achieved good performance, none of them have been compared with clinically used methods for obtaining cerebral hemorrhage volumes. In this paper, the results of segmentation are converted to hemorrhage volume and compared with clinically used methods, demonstrating the great advantages of this method.

3 Dataset

The dataset used in this paper is composed of 341 CT samples that were retrospectively collected from 341 patients of two cohorts that were imaged by GE and Philips CT scan devices between June 2021 and March 2022. All patient-related information was erased. One physician with 5 years of experience delineated the bleeding area slice-by-slice, and another chief physician with 15 years of experience further revised and finalized the data. The background pixels are assigned a value of 0, and the bleeding area is assigned a value of 1. Moreover, the standard windows of 90 Hounsfield units (HU), and center level of 40 HU are employed on all CT samples to limit visual variation. Randomly, the 70%(238) of the 341 CT samples are divided into training sets and 30%(103) into test sets. The training set is used to train the pipeline, and the performance in the test set is used for performance comparation.

The slice number varies from 20 to 47, with the average slice number of 28.13. The height varies from 508 to 512, and the width varies from 508 to 586. The median slice image size is $28 \times 483 \times 483$, with the median spacing as $5 \times 0.518 \times 0.518$ mm^3. The dataset characteristics are shown in Fig. 2.

4 Method

The proposed pipeline is shown in Fig. 3, it is constructed by Pytorch-2.0.0, which takes the 3D CT scans as input and outputs the 3D mask with the same size as input. The pipeline has two key components:1) the cascaded 3D encoder-decoder fully convolutional model to segment hemorrhages from coarse to fine; and 2) the deep supervision mechanism to constrain the training in the intermediate process to speed up model convergence.

4.1 Cascaded 3D Model

The cascaded 3D model is based on the popular encoder-decoder structure, UNet [15], as shown in Fig. 3. It has two stages, the first stage segments the

Item		Train	Test
Patients		239	103
Avg Age		64.05	
Sex	M/F	216/125	
Type	IPH	157 # 65.6%	59 # 57.28%
	IVH	7 # 2.92%	5 # 4.85%
	SAH	36 # 15.06%	15 # 14.56%
	IPH & IVH	39 # 16.31%	24 # 23.30%
Volume (ml)	<30	167 # 69.87%	61 # 59.22%
	30-60	53 # 22.17%	27 # 26.21%
	>60	19 # 7.94%	15 # 14.56%
	min	0.291	0.405
	max	91.97	201.8
	avg	23.452	32.995

Fig. 2. Dataset characteristics. Best view in color.

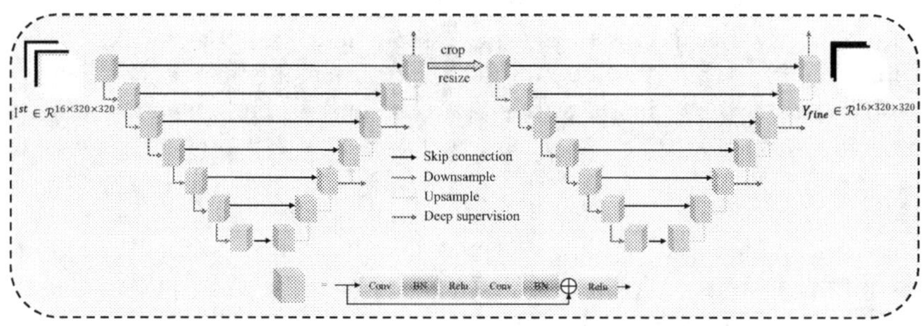

Fig. 3. The diagram of Cascaded Encoder-Decoder convolutional model

coarse bleeding area, and this area is enlarged, cropped, resized, and fed to the second stage to get the precise hemorrhage masks.

The structure of the first stage and the second stage is the same, but weights are not shared. The encoder and decoder both have six levels as shown in Fig. 3, each level has two conv layers, each conv layer is followed by a batch-normalization layer [8] to control gradient explosion and prevent gradient disappearance, and a Relu layer [5] to add more nonlinearity. Moreover, the residual connection [18] is also employed to accelerate gradient propagation. At the same level of the encoder and decoder, the skip connection is used to transfer the low-level texture features lost in the downsampling process to the decoder, which can help the decoder reconstruct high-level semantic features. In the first stage, the cropped CT patch $I_{st} \in \mathcal{R}^{16\times 320\times 320}$ is first sent to the encoder to be downsampled gradually and extract feautres. However, the inter-slice dimension is only downsampled 2 times, and the intra-slice dimension is downsampled 6 times, which generates the bottleneck feature $F_b \in \mathcal{R}^{4\times5\times5}$. Then, F_b is sent to the decoder to upsample and reconstruct the coarse prediction $Y_{coarse} \in \mathcal{R}^{16\times320\times320}$. In the second stage, the coarse bleeding area in Y_{coarse} is cropped and resized as $I_{nd} \in \mathcal{R}^{16\times320\times320}$, which is processed as I_{st} to get the fine prediction $Y_{fine} \in \mathcal{R}^{16\times320\times320}$. Y_{fine} is compared with the label Y_{gt} to calculate the metrics.

4.2 Deep Supervision Mechanism

Deep supervision [9] has been proven to be a plug-and-play technique in training convolutional models, it can regularize the feature extraction and reconstruction of the model and speed up the convergence. Therefore, as the red arrow shown in Fig. 3, we also calculate losses during the upsampling process in the middle, besides the losses in the final predictions in each stage. Then, all these losses are added together to get the final loss. In this work, Dice coefficient (DSC) loss and Cross Entropy (CE) loss are employed in every loss calculation and guide the model to predict more similar results as labels. DSC loss is region-based loss, aims to minimize the mismatch or maximize the overlap region between the label and predicted partition. CE is a distribution-based loss that is designed to minimize the distribution difference between predictions and targets.

4.3 Implementation Details

Convolutional neural networks are data-driven and require large amounts of data to extract semantic information and construct feature representations, so we employed a variety of data augmentation strategies, including: 1) random rotation between −30°C and 30°C; 2) random vertical flipping and horizontal flipping; 3) randomly adding Gaussian noise with 50% probability; 4) random Gaussian smoothing with 50% probability; 5) random contrast adjustment with 50% probability; 6) randomly cropping out a region with a shape of $16 \times 320 \times 320$, where 16 represents the slice depth, and 320×320 indicates the visual size; 7) Normalize the input scan by subtracting the mean value and dividing the standard deviation value. A NVIDIA Tesla A100 (80G) GPU is deployed to run the pipeline, the optimizer is Adamw with the initial learning rate as 1e-2, CosineAnnealingWarmRestarts [12] is used to adjust the learning rate. Dice Similarity Coefficient (DSC) [14], Intersection-over-Union (IOU), Recall, and Precision are used as segmentation evaluation metrics over the testset. In training, we randomly crop input scans to train the pipeline, but the input is orderly cropped into patches with the shape as $16 \times 320 \times 320$ to do the test in the testing phase with the sliding window size as $8 \times 160 \times 160$, and the metrics are calculated after recomposing the ordered patches to the original size, and the overlapped places are averaged.

5 Results

5.1 Ablation Experiment

To show the superior performance of our cascaded model, we set up the following ablation experiment settings: 1) **2D-Model**, this setting has the same structure as the first stage of our cascaded model, except this setting deployed 2D convolution and processed 2D slices with the shape of 512×512 not the sequential scan. 2) **3D-Lowres**, this setting employed the same 3D convolutional structure as the first stage of our cascaded model, but it only had a single stage, and the median voxel size and spacing of the input scan are smaller than our cascaded model, the median voxel size is $28 \times 483 \times 483$, and the spacing is set as $5 \times 0.518 \times 0.518$. 3)**3D-Fullres**, this setting is similar to the **3D-Lowres**, but the median voxel size is $28 \times 512 \times 512$, and the spacing is $5 \times 0.488 \times 0.488$. 4) **3D-Cascaded**, the proposed method in which first stage is the same as **3D-Fullres**, and the second stage is the same as **3D-Lowres**. The experiment results are shown in Table 1.

Table 1. Experiments of segmentation performance

Method	DSC(%)	IOU(%)	Precision(%)	Recall(%)
3D-Cascade	**85.66**	**76.82**	**88.46**	84.11
3D-Fullres	85.19	76.22	88.31	83.54
2D-Model	85.59	76.81	88.04	84.43
3D-Lowres	85.63	76.80	87.83	**84.62**

5.2 Segmentation Accuracy

From the table, we can see that our method achieved the first place in three of the four metrics and obtained overall better results, which shows that compared with the 2D method, the input voxel data allows the network to better capture the contextual information between slices and model the changes in the bleeding region, thus improving the overall segmentation accuracy; and compared with 3D-Fullres and 3D-Lowres, it can be found that the large resolution of volume data can better reveal the details of the bleeding region, thus bringing performance improvement; finally, the 3D-Cascaded employs a two-level segmentation strategy to optimize the segmentation results from coarse to fine, thus achieving a better overall segmentation effect.

$$\mathbb{V}_{MAE} = \frac{\sum_{i}^{N} |V_i - \mathcal{V}_i|}{N} \tag{1}$$

5.3 Diagnostic Accuracy

Among the clinical indicators, the volume of bleeding is a very important factor. We calculate the Mean Absolute Error (MAE) of the bleeding volume between the prediction and GT to compare the diagnostic accuracy, as shown in Eq. 1, where N indicates the number of samples, V and $\mathcal{V}$ represent the volume of the prediction and GT, respectively. The bleeding volume of GT are calculated by ITK-snap [20], while the bleeding volume of prediction is by summing the non-zero pixel number of the prediction mask, and the bleeding volume of prediction is by multiplying the bleeding voxel count and the spacing of the input sample. At present, the most widely used clinical method for measuring bleeding volume is the Tada formula [16,17,19], which was first proposed by Japanese scholars and given as $\frac{\pi}{2 \times A \times B \times C}$, where A (mm) is the maximum bleeding length, B (mm) is the maximum width perpendicular to A (mm) determined on the slice of maximal area, and C is the depth of bleeding, as shown in Fig. 4. For the convenience of clinical practice, the Tada formula is simplified and modified into $\frac{1}{2 \times A \times B \times C}$, which is widely used [3]. Clinically, for IVH and IPH, physicians commonly used the Tada formula method to quickly obtain the hemorrhage volume (ml), while for SAH, due to its scattered and irregular shape, the Tada formula cannot be used to estimate the hemorrhage volume. The experimental results are shown in Table 2. As can be seen, regardless of the experimental configuration, the volume difference for IVH and IPH show a great advantage over the Tada formula, with a minimum improvement of 44.66% and a maximum improvement of 75.54%, obtained by the proposed method. On the volume difference of SAH, the best results were achieved by the proposed method, with an improvement of 49.47%, proving the advantages of the present method. Moreover, our method also has significant advantages in terms of the time required. A physician with 5 years of experience estimated the bleeding volume using the Tada formula in an average of 27.8 s per sample, while our cascaded model predict the bleeding volume in only 6.2 s per sample, which takes only 22.3% of the time of Tada formula, but without losing accuracy.

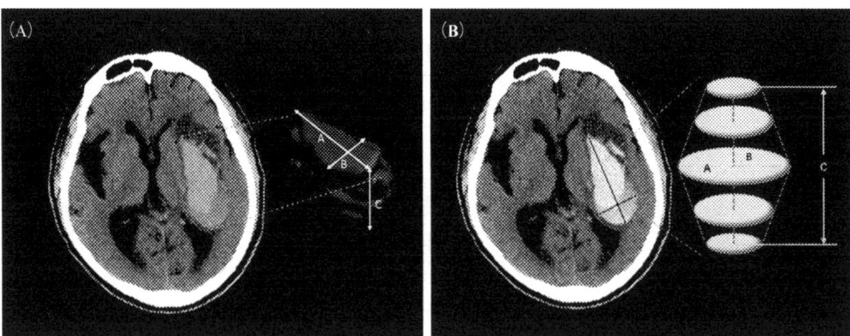

Fig. 4. Display of Tada formula parameters. Best view in color.

Table 2. Diagnostic accuracy comparision, where IPH+IVH+(IPH&IVH) indicates represents the total of these three types of bleeding.

Method	Volume (ml)		Times (s)
-	IPH+IVH+(IPV&IVH)	SAH	-
Tada formula	9.167	-	27.8
2D-Model	5.077	9.298	7.6
3D-Lowres	2.487	5.318	5.7
3D-Fullres	2.442	5.244	5.8
3D-Cascade	2.242	4.698	6.2

6 Conculusions

Our findings indicate that a cascaded encoder-decoder convolutional model can be trained to automatically segment intracranial bleeding in CT images and achieve promising segmentation performance when compared to human experts' hand-contouring reference. These trained cascaded encoder-decoder convolutional models may aid in clinical workflow and allow for more quantitative assessments of CT imaging modalities.

Acknowledgement. This research is supported by the National Key R&D Program of China (Grant No. 2018AAA0102600) and the National Natural Science Foundation of China (Grant No. 62002082).

References

1. Ajoolabady, A., et al.: Targeting autophagy in ischemic stroke: from molecular mechanisms to clinical therapeutics. Pharmacol. Therapeutics 107848 (2021)
2. Donkor, E.S., et al.: Stroke in the century: a snapshot of the burden, epidemiology, and quality of life. Stroke Res. Treat. **2018** (2018)
3. Dsouza, L.B., et al.: Abc/2 estimation in intracerebral hemorrhage: a comparison study between emergency radiologists and emergency physicians. Am. J. Emerg. Med. **37**(10), 1818–1822 (2019)
4. Feng, R., Badgeley, M., Mocco, J., Oermann, E.K.: Deep learning guided stroke management: a review of clinical applications. J. NeuroInterventional Surgery **10**(4), 358–362 (2018). https://doi.org/10.1136/neurintsurg-2017-013355, http://jnis.bmj.com/lookup/doi/10.1136/neurintsurg-2017-013355
5. Glorot, X., Bordes, A., Bengio, Y.: Deep sparse rectifier neural networks. In: Gordon, G.J., Dunson, D.B., Dudík, M. (eds.) Proceedings of the Fourteenth International Conference on Artificial Intelligence and Statistics, AISTATS 2011, Fort Lauderdale, USA, April 11-13, 2011. JMLR Proceedings, vol. 15, pp. 315–323. JMLR.org (2011). http://proceedings.mlr.press/v15/glorot11a/glorot11a.pdf
6. Grewal, M., Srivastava, M.M., Kumar, P., Varadarajan, S.: Radnet: Radiologist level accuracy using deep learning for hemorrhage detection in ct scans. In: 2018 IEEE 15th International Symposium on Biomedical Imaging (ISBI 2018), pp. 281–284 (2018). https://doi.org/10.1109/ISBI.2018.8363574

7. He, X., Chen, K., Hu, K., Chen, Z., Li, X., Gao, X.: Hmoe-net: hybrid multi-scale object equalization network for intracerebral hemorrhage segmentation in CT images. In: Park, T., et al. (eds.) IEEE International Conference on Bioinformatics and Biomedicine, BIBM 2020, Virtual Event, South Korea, 16-19 December 2020, pp. 1006–1009. IEEE (2020). https://doi.org/10.1109/BIBM49941.2020.9313439
8. Ioffe, S., Szegedy, C.: Batch normalization: accelerating deep network training by reducing internal covariate shift. In: International Conference on Machine Learning, pp. 448–456. PMLR (2015)
9. Lee, C., Xie, S., Gallagher, P.W., Zhang, Z., Tu, Z.: Deeply-supervised nets. In: Lebanon, G., Vishwanathan, S.V.N. (eds.) Proceedings of the Eighteenth International Conference on Artificial Intelligence and Statistics, AISTATS 2015, San Diego, California, USA, May 9-12, 2015. JMLR Workshop and Conference Proceedings, vol. 38. JMLR.org (2015). http://proceedings.mlr.press/v38/lee15a.html
10. Lee, J.Y., Kim, J.S., Kim, T.Y., Kim, Y.S.: Detection and classification of intracranial haemorrhage on CT images using a novel deep-learning algorithm. Sci. Rep. **10**(1), 20546 (2020)
11. Lewick, T., Kumar, M., Hong, R., Wu, W.: Intracranial hemorrhage detection in CT scans using deep learning. In: 2020 IEEE Sixth International Conference on Big Data Computing Service and Applications (BigDataService), pp. 169–172. IEEE (2020)
12. Loshchilov, I., Hutter, F.: SGDR: stochastic gradient descent with warm restarts. In: 5th International Conference on Learning Representations, ICLR 2017, Toulon, France, 24–26 April 2017, Conference Track Proceedings. OpenReview.net (2017). https://openreview.net/forum?id=Skq89Scxx
13. Ma, Y., et al.: Iha-net: an automatic segmentation framework for computer-tomography of tiny intracerebral hemorrhage based on improved attention u-net. Biomed. Signal Process. Control **80**, 104320 (2023)
14. Milletari, F., Navab, N., Ahmadi, S.A.: V-net: fully convolutional neural networks for volumetric medical image segmentation. In: 2016 Fourth International Conference on 3D Vision (3DV), pp. 565–571. IEEE (2016)
15. Ronneberger, O., Fischer, P., Brox, T.: U-net: Convolutional networks for biomedical image segmentation. In: International Conference on Medical Image Computing and Computer-Assisted Intervention, pp. 234–241. Springer (2015)
16. Wang, C.W., Juan, C.J., Liu, Y.J., Hsu, H.H., Liu, H.S., Chen, C.Y., Hsueh, C.J., Lo, C.P., Kao, H.W., Huang, G.S.: Volume-dependent overestimation of spontaneous intracerebral hematoma volume by the abc/2 formula. Acta Radiol. **50**(3), 306–311 (2009)
17. Webb, A.J., et al.: Accuracy of the ABC/2 score for intracerebral hemorrhage: systematic review and analysis of MISTIE, CLEAR-IVH, and CLEAR III, and clear iii. Stroke **46**(9), 2470–2476 (2015)
18. Xiao, X., Lian, S., Luo, Z., Li, S.: Weighted res-unet for high-quality retina vessel segmentation. In: 2018 9th International Conference on Information Technology in Medicine and Education (ITME), pp. 327–331 (2018). https://doi.org/10.1109/ITME.2018.00080
19. Xu, X., et al.: Comparison of the tada formula with software slicer: precise and low-cost method for volume assessment of intracerebral hematoma. Stroke **45**(11), 3433–3435 (2014)
20. Yushkevich, P.A., et al.: User-guided 3d active contour segmentation of anatomical structures: significantly improved efficiency and reliability. Neuroimage **31**(3), 1116–1128 (2006). https://doi.org/10.1016/j.neuroimage.2006.01.015

Deep Learning for Ischemic Penumbra Segmentation from MR Perfusion Maps: Robustness to the Deconvolution Algorithm

Theo Leuliet[1(✉)], Stefan Huwer[2], Bénédicte Maréchal[3,4,5], Veronica Ravano[3,4,5], Tobias Kober[3,4,5], Jonathan Rafael-Patiño[4], Johannes Kaesmacher[1], Roland Wiest[1], Jonas Richiardi[4], and Richard McKinley[1]

[1] Support Center for Advanced Neuroimaging, Inselspital, University of Bern, Bern, Switzerland
theocharles.leuliet@insel.ch

[2] Siemens Healthcare GmbH, Erlangen, Germany

[3] Advanced Clinical Imaging Technology, Siemens Healthcare AG, Lausanne, Switzerland

[4] Department of Radiology, Lausanne University Hospital and University of Lausanne, Lausanne, Switzerland

[5] LTS5, École Polytechnique Fédérale de Lausanne (EPFL), Lausanne, Switzerland

Abstract. Determining the penumbra, i.e., the at-risk but salvageable tissue, is crucial in the context of acute ischemic stroke imaging. Deep learning methods performing segmentation from perfusion parameter maps have shown promise in this regard. However, these methods rely on the computation of parameter maps via deconvolution algorithms, raising concerns about their generalizability across different medical centers. This study investigates the robustness of segmentation methods given different perfusion processing algorithms for dynamic susceptibility contrast magnetic resonance perfusion imaging. A neural network is first trained on a dataset of 94 patients with paired Tmax maps from a single MR perfusion algorithm, together with manual perfusion deficit segmentations. The network's outputs are then compared on a second dataset of 268 patients, where Tmax inputs are generated with three different deconvolution algorithms. DICE coefficient along with the difference between estimated perfusion deficit volumes are used to quantify the agreement between predictions. Our findings demonstrate high variability in the predicted penumbra, even when Tmax inputs exhibit high similarity (SSIM $>$ 0.8). This study therefore highlights the importance of exploring deconvolution-free methods to address the robustness issue for learning-based penumbra segmentation.

Keywords: MR Perfusion imaging · Ischemic stroke · Penumbra segmentation · Deep learning

U. Baid et al. (Eds.): BrainLes 2023/SWITCH 2023, LNCS 14668, pp. 106–114, 2024.
https://doi.org/10.1007/978-3-031-76160-7_10

1 Introduction

Ischemic stroke, which accounts for approximately 80% of stroke cases, is a leading cause of disability and mortality worldwide [4]. Accurate prediction of stroke outcomes, as well as the assessment of penumbra, i.e., the at-risk but salvageable tissue, are crucial for effective treatment decision-making [14]. Advancements in medical imaging techniques, specifically Dynamic Susceptibility Contrast (DSC) Magnetic Resonance (MR) perfusion imaging [3], have provided valuable insights into the evaluation of stroke severity.

In clinical routine, a typical estimate for the penumbra is given as the subtraction of the diffusion core from the perfusion deficit. This perfusion deficit is commonly obtained with thresholding methods based on perfusion parameter maps, e.g. time-to-maximum (Tmax), derived from the raw perfusion data [11]. These maps are generated from deconvolution algorithms, which estimate the impulse response of the brain tissue from concentration-time curves of the contrast agent and the arterial input function (AIF).

Recently, classical [8] and deep [2,15] learning methods have shown promising results in performing segmentation using these parameter maps as inputs. However, there are concerns about the robustness of such methods, since deconvolution algorithms, and thus parameter maps, may differ across medical centers. Increasing interest has been observed for deep learning methods that do not rely on parameter maps, especially from computed tomography perfusion (CTP) imaging [12,16]. Learning-based approaches from raw data have also been proposed in magnetic resonance imaging (MRI) [7,18]. The number of such studies is however still limited and these methods do not benefit from the effectiveness of deep learning yet.

The focus of this study is to gain insight on the stability of the perfusion deficit given different MR perfusion processing, and therefore on the need for deconvolution-free learning methods in DSC MR perfusion imaging for ischemic stroke. For this, we evaluate the robustness of a neural network trained on Tmax maps, when applied to another dataset with Tmax maps generated by three different deconvolution algorithms. The findings from this study are expected to contribute to the ongoing efforts in improving ischemic stroke outcome prediction, with the particular interest of having methods that are robust to variations of imaging protocols across different medical centers.

2 Methods

We first obtain a model for delineating the perfusion lesion, which is trained on paired Tmax maps and manual segmentations. In a second step, we consider another dataset consisting of raw MR perfusion data, from which Tmax maps are derived from three different deconvolution algorithms.

2.1 Computation of Tmax

Concentration time curves (CTC) for each voxel can be obtained as

$$CTC(t) = \frac{1}{TE} \log \frac{I(t=0)}{I(t)}, \tag{1}$$

with TE the echo time, $I(t)$ the signal intensity of the voxel at time t. The common model for the concentration time curves can be written as

$$\kappa CTC(t) = CBF \int_0^t AIF(\tau)R(t-\tau)d\tau \tag{2}$$

with κ a constant that depends on hematocrit levels in the arterioles and the density of brain tissue, and the cerebral blood flow (CBF). AIF refers to the arterial input function which is a concentration time curve corresponding to a selected voxel identified as the best representation of the wash-in curve of the contrast agent. The residue function R is the impulse response of the system of neural tissue and vasculature. Tmax corresponds to the time at which R reaches its maximum. The computed residue function for each voxel, and thus the associated Tmax value, mainly depends on two things: the selection of the AIF, and the deconvolution algorithm that is used to retrieve R from the CTC.

2.2 Deconvolution Algorithms

The first considered algorithm corresponds to Olea Sphere's Perfusion MRI oSVD algorithm (OLEA S.A., La Ciotat, France), with automatic AIF selection; we further refer to this method as oSVD. This is the method that is also used during the training phase. We consider two other algorithms that are research applications provided by Siemens Healthineers (Siemens Healthcare, Erlangen, Germany). The first one uses a Tikhonov regularized deconvolution of the AIF from the input signal in Fourier domain [1]. This method is mathematically equivalent to the oSVD [6]; we call it F-oSVD. Note that significant differences can be observed between oSVD and F-oSVD outputs because of their different pre-processing pipelines. The second algorithm uses the circular deconvolution cSVD [17]. Both cSVD and F-oSVD share the same preprocessing pipeline (motion correction, filtering, slice timing correction) as well as the method for the automatic selection of the AIF [10].

2.3 Manual Segmentation of the oSVD Perfusion Maps

The oSVD perfusion maps were manually segmented as part of a previous study [9]: the perfusion lesion apparent on the oSVD-generated Tmax image was manually segmented with the threshold-based brushing tool in Slicer 3D, version 4.8.0 [5] using a Tmax threshold of greater than 4 s.

3 Experiments

3.1 Model Training

To perform the segmentation task from the Tmax maps and manual annotations, we trained a 3D UNET [13].

Training Dataset Description. The dataset used for producing the segmentation model includes 94 patients. We split it into 68 patients for training, 16 for validation and 10 for evaluating the model's performance. The data correspond to sequential cases with MR perfusion from the Swiss Stroke Registry, where an M1 or M2 vessel occlusion is detected. MR acquisitions were performed with a 30 ms echo time and 1400–1610 ms repetition time. Each timepoint has 6–6.5 mm slice thickness; each slice being a 256×256 array with 0.90×0.90 mm^2 in-plane resolution. The number of slices varies between 19 and 23.

From these data, the oSVD algorithm is used to obtain the Tmax maps. Manual segmentation of the perfusion deficit was performed in a two-step manner: a first segmentation was obtained by thresholding the Tmax map to 4 s, then a manual delineation was performed to refine the segmentation.

Network Architecture and Training. The architecture of the convolutional neural network is similar to the UNET in [13], considering 3D convolutions. It has a 5-layer depth, with 32 to 512 feature maps in the encoder pathway. In the first two layers, there is no pooling depth-wise and kernels have a size of $3 \times 3 \times 1$, then pooling is performed across all dimensions and the kernel size is $3 \times 3 \times 3$. In the decoder path, we use 3D transpose convolutions for upsampling.

Before being fed to the network, Tmax maps are interpolated to have a 6.5 mm slice thickness. Zero-padding is performed when needed to get 19 slices for all the volumes. Then, Tmax maps are clipped between 0 and 10 s. Finally downsampling to 128×128 slices with 1.8×1.8 mm^2 voxel size is performed.

We use DICE loss and ADAM optimizer for training, with a learning rate of 10^{-3}. We train the parameters for 200 epochs, and we save the model from the epoch that achieves the best DICE validation metric. Training takes approximately 10 min, while inference takes around 0.4 s. Computations are performed on a NVIDIA RTX A6000 with 48GB GPU memory.

On the 10 test volumes from this 94-patient dataset, we obtain a DICE of 0.828, a value for the Area Under the Curve (AUC) of 0.978, a mean absolute error for the computed perfusion deficit volume of 16.85 ml, corresponding to a mean relative error of 12.2%.

3.2 Data for the Study

The dataset that we use for the robustness evaluation also comes from the Swiss Stroke Registry, but the selection criteria is different compared to the training set: these are sequential cases with MR perfusion where there is either anterior or middle cerebral artery occlusion. It has a total of 268 patients, none of which are part of the 94 patient-dataset used during the training stage. Acquisitions were performed with a 30 ms echo time and 1400–1700 ms repetition time, i.e., comparable to the protocol used for the training data. The number of slices varies between 19 and 25. All slices are 256×256 with 0.90×0.90 mm^2 in-plane resolution. Slice thickness ranges from 6 to 6.5 mm. We apply all three perfusion algorithms to this dataset, and then apply the segmentation algorithm, resampling the Tmax maps to match the dimension of the inputs given to the network during the training phase.

3.3 Method for Evaluation

For this dataset we have no manual delineation of the perfusion deficit volume. The evaluation therefore consists in comparing the different model outputs with each other, depending on the deconvolution algorithm. We use the DICE coefficient as well as the volume absolute error (VAE), i.e., the absolute difference between the total segmented volume (in ml) obtained with two different methods. Before computing metrics or showing visualizations, we set to 0 all voxels for which the Tmax value is under 6 s, which allows to further refine the model output. To assess the similarity of the inputs of the network, we compute the Structural Similarity Index Measure (SSIM) between Tmax values that are clipped between 0 and 10 s.

4 Results and Discussion

4.1 Quantitative Comparison

Mean values for SSIM, DICE and VAE are shown in Table 1. Overall, DICE and VAE values seem to show differences between the predicted segmentations. Predictions from F-oSVD and cSVD are the ones that have the highest mismatch in terms of DICE (0.418) and VAE (37.98 ml). Their corresponding Tmax maps

Table 1. SSIM between Tmax maps, DICE and Volume absolute error (VAE) in ml between different predictions depending on the deconvolution algorithm.

SSIM	cSVD	oSVD
F-oSVD	0.724 ± 0.042	0.689 ± 0.046
cSVD	x	0.771 ± 0.054
DICE	cSVD	oSVD
F-oSVD	0.418 ± 0.291	0.431 ± 0.293
cSVD	x	0.578 ± 0.286
VAE	cSVD	oSVD
F-oSVD	37.98 ± 33.70	32.79 ± 34.15
cSVD	x	17.67 ± 26.75

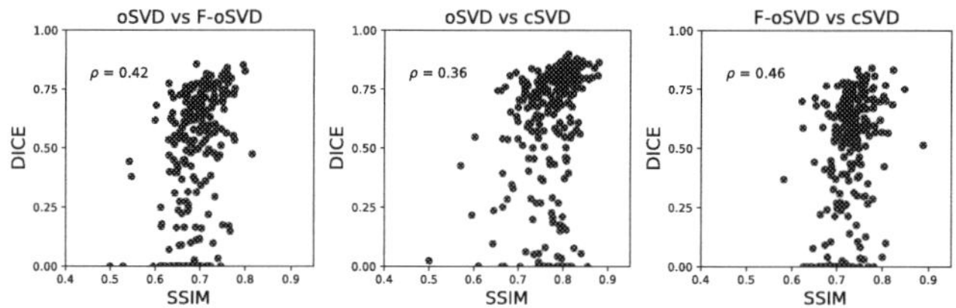

Fig. 1. SSIM vs DICE scatter plots for each pair of methods.

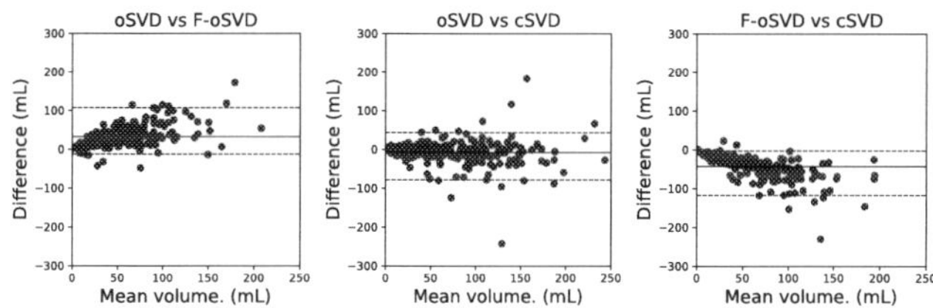

Fig. 2. Bland-Altman plots for each pair of methods.

have the second least similarity with each other as assessed by the 0.724 mean SSIM value. For both cSVD and oSVD algorithms, the lowest SSIM for Tmax is obtained when compared to F-oSVD. Interestingly, this is also the case for the lowest DICE and the highest volume absolute error.

This observation suggests that the similarity between two segmentations is dependent on the similarity between the corresponding Tmax inputs. We investigate this hypothesis by plotting the DICE value depending on the SSIM value of the Tmax maps, for each pair of methods, in Fig. 1. Correlation is observed between SSIM and DICE values, but the Spearman coefficient ranges from $\rho = 0.36$ to $\rho = 0.46$ depending on the pair. This shows that even if two Tmax maps are similar to each other, this might not be the case for the corresponding segmentation. Indeed, in Fig. 1 we observe some cases where the SSIM is above 0.800 and the corresponding DICE is below 0.1. This observation is an argument for the lack of robustness of the predictive model.

4.2 Qualitative Assessment of Segmentations

Representative examples from the evaluation dataset are shown in Fig. 3. As can be seen, the segmented perfusion mask differs substantially between algorithms. In general, for all methods there are regions with elevated Tmax (>6 s) within the hypoperfusion which are not included in the segmentation: the oSVD-generated Tmax map exhibits this least, which is unsurprising given that this method was used to generate training data. However, we see substantial underestimation of the hypoperfused area volume on Patient 3, along with some false positive voxels on the contralateral hemisphere.

F-oSVD maps show less hypoperfused tissue in general, but we also observe underestimation of the perfusion deficit volume within the segmentation when

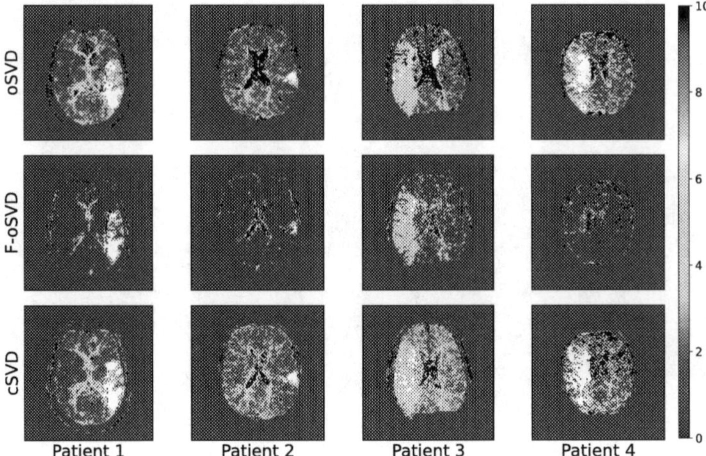

Fig. 3. Estimated perfusion lesion (in white) depending on the perfusion algorithm. The colorbar is in seconds, and Tmax maps are clipped to 10 s.

compared to visual assessment. There are more visible hypoperfused voxels on cSVD Tmax maps, and thus a larger segmented area as compared to F-oSVD, but in this case also there seems to be some underestimation of the perfusion deficit volume.

Bland-Altman plots in Fig. 2 highlight the high number of cases for which there is a strong mismatch between the estimated perfusion deficit volume. In most of those cases, large volume differences result from one deconvolution algorithm producing a poor-quality Tmax map where hypoperfused areas are less distinguishable, like it is the case for Patient 4.

Overall, we observe that DSC perfusion processing can lead to poor-quality Tmax maps, for which the segmentation model cannot retrieve the right voxels belonging to the hypoperfused area. We also observe that the F-oSVD and cSVD algorithms differ substantially in the produced segmentation while sharing the same preprocessing and AIF inference. This emphasizes the already known issue of consistency between different deconvolution algorithms, especially considering that the problem (2) is ill-posed.

A major observation from this study is that even when the deconvolution algorithm generates Tmax maps that are quantitatively similar - as assessed with SSIM -, the segmentation model might generate significantly different perfusion deficit areas. This questions the method itself that consists in predicting this perfusion deficit with trained neural networks on the basis of perfusion maps. A solution could be to include Tmax maps from different deconvolution methods in the training set, but this can be impractical and there are many different pipelines for parameter maps generation across different centers. This work therefore encourages research towards deep learning-based methods from parameter maps that are specifically designed to be robust to the deconvolution algorithm. Another possibility might be to have methods that are deconvolution free. Neural networks that directly map the source perfusion data to the perfusion lesion segmentation, as it has been proposed for CT perfusion imaging [12,16], might in this sense be an interesting solution to investigate.

5 Conclusion

The purpose of the study was to assess the robustness of a trained neural network when the input Tmax maps are generated by different deconvolution algorithms. Our results show high variability in the predicted perfusion lesion segmentations. We observe that artefacts on Tmax maps give poor segmentation outcomes. More important, we find that similar inputs can lead to large mismatches on the predictions. This study suggests that this field of research could benefit from deconvolution-free segmentation methods.

References

1. Calamante, F., Gadian, D.G., Connelly, A.: Quantification of bolus-tracking MRI: improved characterization of the tissue residue function using Tikhonov regularization. Magnetic Resonance in Medicine: An Official Journal of the International Society for Magnetic Resonance in Medicine **50**(6), 1237–1247 (2003)
2. Clerigues, A., et al.: Acute ischemic stroke lesion core segmentation in CT perfusion images using fully convolutional neural networks. Comput. Biol. Med. **115**, 103487 (2019)
3. Copen, W.A., Schaefer, P.W., Wu, O.: MR Perfusion Imaging in Acute Ischemic Stroke. Neuroimaging Clin. N. Am. **21**(2), 259–283 (2011)
4. Donkor, E.S.: Stroke in the century: a snapshot of the burden, epidemiology, and quality of life. Stroke research and treatment **2018** (2018)
5. Fedorov, A., et al.: 3D Slicer as an image computing platform for the Quantitative Imaging Network. Magn. Reson. Imaging **30**(9), 1323–1341 (2012)
6. Gall, P., et al.: On the design of filters for Fourier and oSVD-based deconvolution in bolus tracking perfusion MRI. Magn. Reson. Mater. Phys., Biol. Med. **23**, 187–195 (2010)
7. Ho, K.C.: Predicting ischemic stroke tissue fate using a deep convolutional neural network on source magnetic resonance perfusion images. J. Med. Imag. **6**(02), 1 (2019)
8. McKinley, R., et al.: A Machine Learning Approach to Perfusion Imaging With Dynamic Susceptibility Contrast MR. Front. Neurol. **9**, 717 (2018)
9. Meier, R., et al.: Neural network–derived perfusion maps for the assessment of lesions in patients with acute ischemic stroke. Radiology: artificial intelligence **1**(5), e190019 (2019)
10. Mouridsen, K., et al.: Automatic selection of arterial input function using cluster analysis. Magn. Reson. Med. **55**(3), 524–531 (2006)
11. Olivot, J.M., et al.: Geography, structure, and evolution of diffusion and perfusion lesions in diffusion and perfusion imaging evaluation for understanding stroke evolution (defuse). Stroke **40**(10), 3245–3251 (2009)
12. Robben, D., et al.: Prediction of final infarct volume from native CT perfusion and treatment parameters using deep learning. Medical Image Analysis **59** (Jan 2020)

13. Ronneberger, O., Fischer, P., Brox, T.: U-net: Convolutional networks for biomedical image segmentation. In: Medical Image Computing and Computer-Assisted Intervention–MICCAI 2015: 18th International Conference, Munich, Germany, October 5-9, 2015, Proceedings, Part III 18. pp. 234–241. Springer (2015)
14. Schlaug, G., et al.: The ischemic penumbra: operationally defined by diffusion and perfusion MRI. Neurology **53**(7), 1528–1528 (1999)
15. Wang, G., et al.: Automatic ischemic stroke lesion segmentation from computed tomography perfusion images by image synthesis and attention-based deep neural networks. Med. Image Anal. **65**, 101787 (2020)
16. Winder, A.J., et al.: Predicting the tissue outcome of acute ischemic stroke from acute 4D computed tomography perfusion imaging using temporal features and deep learning. Front. Neurosci. **16**, 1009654 (2022)
17. Wu, O., et al.: Tracer arrival timing-insensitive technique for estimating flow in MR perfusion-weighted imaging using singular value decomposition with a block-circulant deconvolution matrix. Magn. Reson. Med. **50**(1), 164–174 (2003)
18. Yu, Y., et al.: Prediction of Hemorrhagic Transformation Severity in Acute Stroke From Source Perfusion MRI. IEEE Trans. Biomed. Eng. **65**(9), 2058–2065 (2018)

From Brain Tissue Infarction at 24 Hours to Patient Functional Outcome at 90 Days Using Deep Learning

Marie Ulens(✉), Jeroen Bertels, Ewout Heylen, Julie Lambert, Jelle Demeestere, Robin Lemmens, Dirk Vandermeulen, and Frederik Maes

KU Leuven, Leuven, Belgium
marie.ulens@outlook.com, frederik.maes@kuleuven.be

Abstract. Accurate functional outcome prediction shortly after the onset of stroke would enable more effective personalized care of stroke patients. A deep learning approach was developed that utilizes follow-up images at 24 h to predict the functional outcome 90 days after stroke onset. The method involves the use of a conventional U-net segmentation model that was trained to delineate the stroke lesion on CT images, with an additional branch integrated into the U-net's bottom layer to extract features for a separately trained network that classifies cases into favorable (modified Rankin Score (mRS) = 0–2) or unfavorable outcomes (mRS = 3–6). The method was trained and validated using 3-fold cross-validation on a set of 240 images (training: 170; validation: 90). The lesion segmentation yielded an average Dice score of 0.458 and an average absolute volume error of 10.71 ml, while the binary mRS prediction obtained an overall accuracy of 88.6% on the training set and 58.0% on the validation set. Although there is much room for improvement, these results demonstrate the potential of deep learning approaches toward a promising decision-support tool for stroke outcome prediction.

Keywords: Ischemic stroke · Deep learning · Outcome prediction

1 Introduction

An ischemic stroke, or brain tissue infarction, occurs when the blood supply to part of the brain is blocked, leading to potentially long-lasting brain damage, disability, and, in extreme cases, death [1]. The global burden of stroke has increased significantly between 1990 and 2019, according to the Global Stroke Fact Sheet of 2022 [7]. Therefore, implementing innovative techniques, such as functional outcome prediction, is essential to mitigate this burden by enabling clinicians to administer personalized stroke care. Moreover, quick determination of the most suitable treatment saves time and money for patients, clinicians, and hospitals and optimizes the allocation of healthcare and social resources [8]. Lin et al. emphasize that more realistic recovery and rehabilitation goals can be

U. Baid et al. (Eds.): BrainLes 2023/SWITCH 2023, LNCS 14668, pp. 115–123, 2024.
https://doi.org/10.1007/978-3-031-76160-7_11

set, enhancing shared after-care decisions and improving expectation management [11]. Consequently, the ultimate goal is to develop a functional outcome prediction model that achieves a sufficiently high accuracy ensuring its reliability as a decision-support tool in clinical practice. Function outcome in stroke is typically evaluated using the Modified Rankin Scale for Neurologic Disability (mRS), which measures the degree of disability or dependence on the daily activities of the patient.

Deep learning using Convolutional Neural Networks (CNN) has proven to be successful in medical imaging segmentation and classification tasks and has also been applied for stroke lesion segmentation and outcome prediction. Bacchi *et al.* [2] reported an Area Under the Curve (AUC) of 0.75 for functional outcome prediction by combining a CNN with an Artificial Neural Network (ANN). The CNN was employed for feature extraction from non-contrast-enhanced computed tomography (CT) scans, while the ANN performed classification based on clinical data. Similarly, Choi *et al.* [5] used a CNN as a feature extractor alongside a shallow neural network comprising fully-connected layers for multi-class mRS prediction. For brain image segmentation, the U-net architecture is widely employed. Nielsen *et al.* [12] built and trained their own CNNs based on the U-net design, achieving an AUC of 0.88 ± 0.12 for predicting the outcome in acute ischemic stroke patients. Another variant of U-net for (chronic) stroke lesion segmentation was proposed by Zhou *et al.* [16] incorporating 2D and 3D convolution kernels through a dimension transform block to combine the benefits of both approaches. Omarov *et al.* [14] published a modified U-net model that utilized simple techniques such as data augmentation, L2 regularization, and dropout to enhance segmentation performance. They achieved a Dice score of 0.58, establishing themselves as state-of-the-art for stroke lesion segmentation. Furthermore, Nishi *et al.* [13] proposed a two-output deep learning model based on an encoder-decoder CNN architecture for segmentation, achieving comparable Dice scores on their validation set. Ding *et al.* [6] introduced a model that outperformed all state-of-the-art methods, reaching a Dice score of 0.91 for the segmentation and an accuracy of 0.975 for outcome prediction. However, these results should be considered in the context of an extensive dataset of almost 1500 patients and a significant class imbalance of 87.7% to 12.3%. Their approach combined various state-of-the-art techniques to construct a model solely based on 14 deep neuroimaging features extracted from CNNs.

In this paper, a novel two-output deep learning model is proposed, offering unique advantages compared to state-of-the-art approaches: Unlike most existing methods, both segmentation and classification are integrated into a single model architecture, utilizing deep learning features extracted from the segmentation for outcome prediction. Additionally, the model uses CT images, which are more widely available in healthcare facilities, providing a broad applicability of the model. Specifically, the use of dual-energy CT scans allows for enhanced tissue characterization and improved image quality. Another notable feature is the utilization of follow-up images rather than acute phase images, which provides a clearer view of the infarcted tissue by minimizing the presence of penumbra volume. Moreover, during the initial twelve hours of an ischemic stroke, the stroke region may not be readily visible on a CT scan due to collateral circulation, which can temporarily compensate for the blocked blood supply. However, after 12–24 hours, in the follow-up phase, the brain region experiencing reduced or no blood flow becomes hypodense, making the stroke lesion visible on a CT scan. Lastly, the model's ability to predict the mRS without relying on clinical metadata enhances its accessibility by promoting model simplicity, overcoming difficulties related to obtaining complete metadata, and facilitating generalization to diverse settings where such metadata might not be easily accessible.

2 Methods

2.1 Patient Data

The KAROLINSKA dataset originates from the Karolinska University Hospital in Sweden and includes follow-up Dual-Energy Non-Contrast CT (DENCCT) scans with a voxel size of 1.5mm, acquired from 510 patients [10]. An experienced neurologist and neuroradiologist manually delineated these brain images, leveraging their DE character, to create a reference stroke segmentation for training the deep learning model. Furthermore, an inter-observer Dice coefficient of 0.49 and an inter-observer volume error of 18.1ml were calculated for these delineations by both experts, as reported in Heylen *et al.* [9]. No specific techniques were employed to further exploit the DE character of the images during the model's training process. In addition, the dataset contains the corresponding clinical metadata and the mRS three months post-stroke. The modified Rankin Scale (mRS) is a widely-used measure to evaluate stroke recovery [3]. The scale uses a seven-category classification system, ranging from 0 (no symptoms) to 6 (dead). The mRS score is binarized by merging the seven mRS categories into two groups: patients with a favorable (mRS = 0–2) and patients with an unfavorable outcome (mRS=3–6). Due to various limitations affecting certain scans, including insufficient spatial and temporal resolution, motion artifacts, limited contrast, corrupted files, and the absence of brain and lesion images [9], only 385 patient files were preserved.

Moreover, patients with missing mRS values were excluded, leaving 260 cases available for training the CNN. The KAROLINSKA dataset is well-balanced, with 53% favorable and 47% unfavorable outcomes. It was ensured that a similar balance was maintained in all folds during cross-validation training of the deep learning approaches.

2.2 Deep Learning Architecture

A two-output U-net model, depicted in Fig. 1, was developed, with one output being the lesion segmentation of the brain image, while the second output is the prediction of the (binary) mRS. The model was implemented as a KerasModel transformer using the DeepVoxNet2 package [4]. The U-net architecture consists of four levels of convolutional layers, each comprising multiple 3D convolutional operations to extract deep learning features from the input image.

Each convolutional operation is preceded by an instance normalization step and employs a Leaky ReLU activation function. The model takes an input image of size $81 \times 81 \times 81 \times 1$ and produces a $3 \times 3 \times 3 \times 120$ feature vector in its deepest layer while the expanding path generates high-resolution segmentation images. The expanding and contracting paths are connected through concatenating layers to preserve spatial information. The final layer of the U-net yields the lesion segmentation output, denoted as S0, with dimensions $81 \times 81 \times 81 \times 1$. An additional branch is integrated into the bottom layer of the U-net. This branch aims to train the model for outcome prediction by using the extracted deep-learning features from the segmentation network and the downsampled segmentation result, leveraging spatial information to potentially improve the mRS prediction. A 3D convolutional operation is applied to downsample the feature maps to a dimension of $1 \times 1 \times 1 \times 60$. Subsequently, two fully connected layers with 'softmax' activation and a dropout layer, to prevent overfitting, are utilized to produce the classification output, denoted as S1, with dimensions $1 \times 1 \times 1 \times 2$. The lesion volume is derived from the segmentation output S0, while output S1 is converted into a binary integer representing either a favorable or unfavorable outcome.

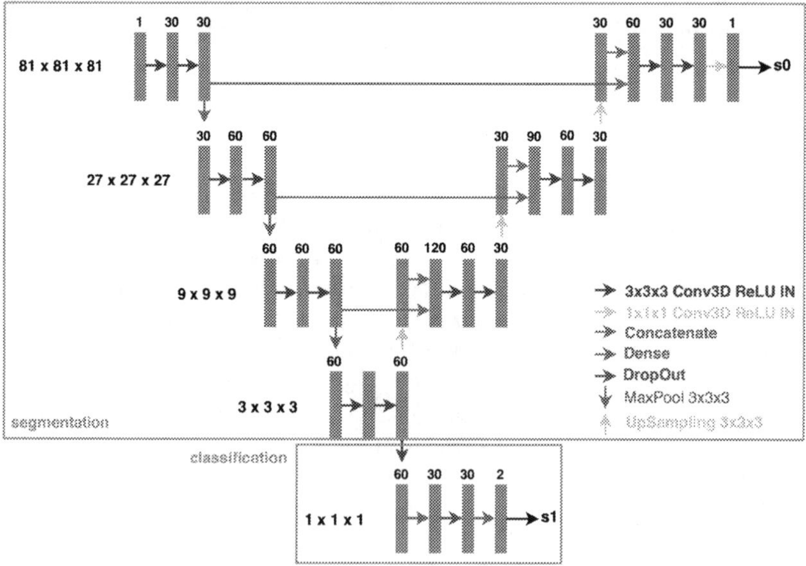

Fig. 1. Two-output U-net model trained for stroke lesion segmentation (green) and functional outcome prediction (orange) of DENCCT images. (Color figure online)

2.3 Training

The U-net was trained using three-fold cross-validation. Each fold includes a training set of approximately 170 cases, while the validation set comprises around 90 patients. Data augmentation of the training set was applied by transforming the original DENCCT images through affine deformation, normalization, and flipping. The images were centrally cropped to the input size of $81 \times 81 \times 81$ voxels based on brain image masks. In order to train the two-output U-net model efficiently, a two-step training approach was implemented. In the first round, the entire model was trained for segmentation, assigning a weight of 1 to output S0 and 0 to output S1. The U-net was trained for, on average, 184 epochs, optimizing both cross-entropy and Dice loss functions simultaneously with equal weights. The training was conducted using a batch size of 4 and an initial learning rate of 1e–3. In the second round, only the additional bottom branch was trained for classification, assigning a weight of 0 to S0 and 1 to S1. It was trained for 210 epochs on average, using the cross-entropy loss function while employing a batch size of 8 and an initial learning rate of 1e–5. These hyperparameters were fine-tuned based on the first fold. In addition, early stopping was implemented during training, and L2 regularization was introduced to discourage overfitting. The final model was selected based on its best performance on both the validation and training sets. Note that the decision not to train both tasks simultaneously with non-zero weights for both S0 and S1 was influenced by computational limitations, concerns about potential interference, and optimization challenges. Although, in future research, it could be interesting to investigate the impact of simultaneous training with a combined loss function after the two initial training tasks or as an alternative approach.

3 Results

3.1 Lesion Segmentation

The performance of the segmentation model is presented in Table 1, demonstrating the Dice score and the absolute volume difference. The training set yields a favorable Dice score of 0.752, while the validation set achieves a lower Dice score of 0.458, indicating potential overfitting despite the measures taken during model selection. Similarly, the absolute volume difference may be affected by overfitting, as it is minimal for the training set (1.24 ml) but higher for the validation set (10.71 ml). Table 2 provides a comprehensive context on the volume error results.

Examples of the stroke lesion segmentation in a patient with a favorable outcome (mRS = 2) and a patient with an unfavorable outcome (mRS=5) are illustrated in Fig. 2. The yellow-colored tissue depicts the manual stroke segmentation conducted by an experienced neurologist and neuroradiologist, while the underlying red color represents the lesion segmentation predicted by the U-net model. A visual inspection reveals that both the manual and predicted segmentation exhibit similar shapes in the axial and coronal planes. However, upon closer

Table 1. Segmentation performance of the U-net model, trained with 3-fold cross-validation.

	Dice score	Volume error
Training	0.752	1.24 ml
Validation	0.458	10.71 ml

Table 2. Descriptive statistics of the true stroke volumes in the dataset.

Mean	47.89 ml
Standard deviation	82.21 ml
Maximum	663.28 ml
Third quartile	56.96 ml
Median	14.90 ml
First quartile	3.00 ml
Minimum	0.00 ml

examination, it becomes evident that the predicted segmentation tends to underestimate the actual lesion volume. Furthermore, a visual comparison between the favorable and unfavorable cases demonstrates that the predicted stroke volume (red) appears slightly larger for the unfavorable outcome, whereas the true stroke volume (yellow) remains relatively similar for both outcomes. This observation implies that the U-net model associates a larger stroke volume with an unfavorable outcome, although this notion is not confirmed by the true volumes. Moreover, this remark is consistently observed in all predicted cases and is not limited to the cases illustrated in this paper.

3.2 mRS Prediction

The binary classification results on the validation dataset, utilizing deep learning features extracted from the brain images, are summarized in Table 3. The model correctly classifies the majority of the cases, achieving an overall accuracy of 58.0%. Moreover, it demonstrates a sensitivity of 47.6%, a specificity of 69.0%, and an F1-score of 53.5% when utilizing a classification threshold of 0.5. This threshold was chosen based on a scatter plot representing the relationship between the classification threshold and the prediction outputs. Furthermore, an average AUC of 0.627 is obtained. Notably, a higher accuracy of 68.9% is achieved on the validation set of the first fold, on which the model was primarily optimized. In comparison, the second and third fold obtained lower accuracies of 55.1% and 50.0%, respectively. Additionally, it should be highlighted that an overall training accuracy of 88.6% was achieved, suggesting significant overfitting but also indicating the potential of the U-net model. Finally, it should be remarked that performing the classification without the segmentation pretraining of the model results in worse prediction performance, indicating the added value of using the complete U-net model.

4 Discussion

The performance of the segmentation model in this study is consistent with findings from related studies. For instance, Ronneberger *et al.* achieved a Dice score of 0.46 using their original 5-level U-net segmentation model [14,15]. Notably,

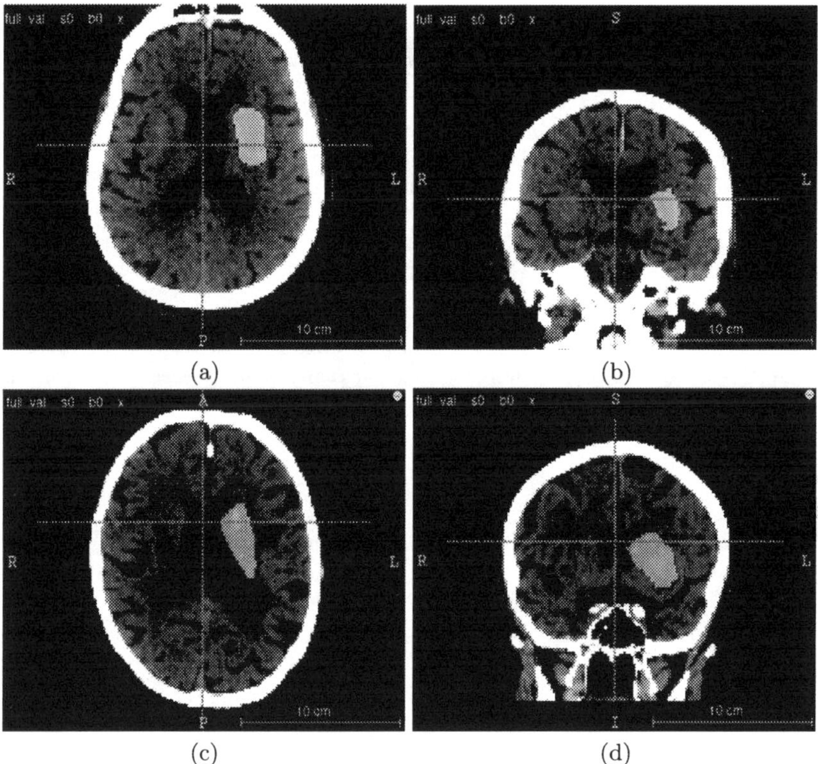

Fig. 2. Visual representation of the manual (yellow) and predicted (red) stroke lesion segmentation in DENCCT brain image of a patient with a favorable outcome (mRS = 2) (a, b) and a patient with an unfavorable outcome (mRS = 5) (c, d). (Color figure online)

Omarov *et al.* introduced modifications to the classical U-net architecture that were also employed in this study but reached a superior Dice score of 0.58 [14]. This improvement can potentially be attributed to the inclusion of a fifth level of layers. Similarly to the U-net in this paper, Nishi *et al.* utilized a two-output U-net model with four levels of convolutional layers [13]. Compared to the performance of our model, they obtained a slightly higher Dice score of 0.58 ± 0.01 on the validation set, whereas a lower Dice score of 0.63 ± 0.01 was achieved on the training set. Since the dataset has a mean stroke volume of 47.89ml, the low Dice score cannot be attributed to small lesion volumes. For the mRS prediction, Nishi *et al.* reported an accuracy of 65.4%, a sensitivity of 72.2%, and a specificity of 60.2%, which is slightly higher than the proposed model. However, they obtained a significantly lower training accuracy of 72.4% compared to the 88.6% training accuracy in this study, suggesting that their model may have superior generalizability.

Table 3. Outcome prediction performance of the U-net model, trained with 3-fold cross-validation.

	Accuracy	Sensitivity	Specificity	F1-score	AUC
U-net model	**0.580**	0.476	0.690	0.535	0.627
	Fold 1	Fold 2	Fold 3	Average	
Accuracy	0.689	0.551	0.500	**0.580**	

Finally, it is important to emphasize that the training of the U-net model in this study was optimized exclusively on the first fold, leading to lower performances on the second and third fold and, consequently, decreasing the average performance. The optimized hyperparameters, including batch size, learning rate, number of epochs, data augmentation extent, sample shuffling per epoch, loss weights, regularization parameters, and model architecture, have a significant impact on the classification performance. Therefore, further research is necessary to refine these hyperparameters across all three folds and to enhance generalizability.

5 Conclusion

The presented deep learning model demonstrates notable performance in accurately segmenting and classifying functional outcomes based solely on DENCCT images, positioning itself among state-of-the-art models in this field. Its uniqueness lies in the integration of both segmentation and classification within a single model and the utilization of DENCCT follow-up images. While there is ample room for improvement in both tasks, this research study emphasizes the potential and feasibility of this technique. An important limitation of the current study is overfitting, addressing this issue would enhance the model's accuracy performance, generalizability, and robustness in mRS prediction. Additionally, if future advancements prove insufficient, the exploration of incorporating metadata or using combined approaches should be considered.

Acknowledgements. We want to express our sincere gratitude to Fredrik Ståhl and Åke Holmberg for providing the KAROLINSKA dataset, which has been instrumental in facilitating our research endeavors.

References

1. Stroke. Mayo Clinic. https://www.mayoclinic.org/diseases-conditions/stroke/symptoms-causes/syc-20350113, last checked on 12 May 2023, https://www.mayoclinic.org/diseases-conditions/stroke/symptoms-causes/syc-20350113
2. Bacchi, S., Zerner, T., Oakden-Rayner, L., Kleinig, T., Patel, S., Jannes, J.: Deep learning in the prediction of ischaemic stroke thrombolysis functional outcomes: a pilot study. Acad. Radiol. **27**, e19–e23 (2020). https://doi.org/10.1016/j.acra.2019.03.015

3. Banks, J.L., Marotta, C.A.: Outcomes validity and reliability of the modified rankin scale: implications for stroke clinical trials - a literature review and synthesis. Stroke **38**, 1091–1096 (2007). https://doi.org/10.1161/01.STR.0000258355.23810.c6
4. Bertels, J., Robben, D., Lemmens, R., Vandermeulen, D.: DeepVoxNet2: yet another CNN framework, November 2022. http://arxiv.org/abs/2211.09569
5. Choi, Y., Kwon, Y., Lee, H., Kim, B.J., Paik, M.C., Won, J.H.: Ensemble of deep convolutional neural networks for prognosis of ischemic stroke, pp. 231–243 (2016)
6. Ding, L., Liu, Z., Mane, R., Wang, S., Jing, J., et al., H.F.: Predicting functional outcome in patients with acute brainstem infarction using deep neuroimaging features. Eur. J. Neurol. **29**, 744–752 (2022). https://doi.org/10.1111/ene.15181
7. Feigin, V.L., Brainin, M., Norrving, B., Martins, S., Sacco, R.L., et al., W.H.: World stroke organization (WSO): global stroke fact sheet 2022, November 2022. https://doi.org/10.1177/17474930211065917
8. Goyal, M., Ospel, J.M., Kappelhof, M., Ganesh, A.: Challenges of outcome prediction for acute stroke treatment decisions. Stroke 1921–1928 (2021). https://doi.org/10.1161/STROKEAHA.120.033785
9. Heylen, E., Vandermeulen, D., Maes, F., Dupont, P., Scheldeman, L., Lambert, J., Bertels, J.: Modelling the evolution of brain tissue status in ischemic stroke using CNNs. Master thesis, KU Leuven (2021)
10. Karolinska University Hospital. https://www.karolinska.se/en/karolinska-university-hospital/
11. Lin, C.H., Hsu, K.C., Johnson, K.R., Fann, Y.C., Tsai, C.H., et al., Y.S.: Evaluation of machine learning methods to stroke outcome prediction using a nationwide disease registry. Comput. Methods Program. Biomed. **190** (2020). https://doi.org/10.1016/j.cmpb.2020.105381
12. Nielsen, A., Hansen, M.B., Tietze, A., Mouridsen, K.: Prediction of tissue outcome and assessment of treatment effect in acute ischemic stroke using deep learning. Stroke **49**, 1394–1401 (2018). https://doi.org/10.1161/STROKEAHA.117.019740
13. Nishi, H., et al.: Deep learning-derived high-level neuroimaging features predict clinical outcomes for large vessel occlusion. Stroke 1484–1492 (2020). https://doi.org/10.1161/STROKEAHA.119.028101
14. Omarov, B., et al.: Modified unet model for brain stroke lesion segmentation on computed tomography images. Comput. Mater. Continua **71**, 4701–4717 (2022). https://doi.org/10.32604/cmc.2022.020998
15. Ronneberger, O., Fischer, P., Brox, T.: U-net: convolutional networks for biomedical image segmentation, pp. 234–241 (2015)
16. Zhou, Y., Huang, W., Dong, P., Xia, Y., Wang, S.: D-unet: a dimension-fusion u shape network for chronic stroke lesion segmentation, August 2019. https://doi.org/10.1109/TCBB.2019.2939522, http://arxiv.org/abs/1908.05104

Functional Outcome Prediction in Acute Ischemic Stroke

Ewout Heylen[1(✉)], Jeroen Bertels[1], Julie Lambert[1], Jelle Demeestere[1], Fredrik Ståhl[2], Åke Holmberg[2], Wim van Zwam[3], Charles Majoie[4], Aad van der Lugt[5], Robin Lemmens[1], and Frederik Maes[1]

[1] KU Leuven, Leuven, Belgium
ewout.heylen@kuleuven.be
[2] Karolinska Institutet, Stockholm, Sweden
[3] Maastricht UMC, Maastricht, The Netherlands
[4] Amsterdam UMC, Amsterdam, The Netherlands
[5] Erasmus MC, Rotterdam, The Netherlands

Abstract. BACKGROUND Stroke is one of the most prevalent neurological diseases and causes of disability worldwide. Functional outcome prediction models can assist the treatment decision process and optimize acute ischemic stroke health care. Current models often use a limited set of input features to predict functional outcome, although combining various types of features could improve model performance. Furthermore, they often incorporate follow-up information, while prediction models applicable in the acute setting are desirable. METHODS We trained an ensemble model consisting of five machine learning models with leave-one-out cross-validation to predict the binarized modified Rankin Scale score three months after stroke onset in patients with acute ischemic stroke caused by a large vessel occlusion who received endovascular treatment. We used clinical variables, treatment variables and lesion loads derived from registration of a stroke population-specific neuroanatomical CT brain atlas with the follow-up non-contrast enhanced CT scan as input features. RESULTS Taking into account five performance metrics (accuracy, AUC, sensitivity, specificity and F1-score), the ensemble model and support vector machine (SVM) seemed to achieve the best performances out of the six models (ensemble model and the five individual machine learning models), with AUC values up to 0.76 and 0.77 respectively. The highest accuracy obtained with the ensemble model was 0.69, and with the SVM 0.72. Little variance in performance was found between the various sets of input features. CONCLUSION Although similar performances compared to current literature were obtained, conventional machine learning models might not be sophisticated enough to capture the complex interactions between input features for functional outcome prediction in acute ischemic stroke.

Keywords: Acute ischemic stroke · Functional outcome prediction · Machine learning

U. Baid et al. (Eds.): BrainLes 2023/SWITCH 2023, LNCS 14668, pp. 124–133, 2024.
https://doi.org/10.1007/978-3-031-76160-7_12

1 Introduction

Stroke is one of the most prevalent neurological diseases and causes of disability worldwide. In the EU, 1.12 million cases were reported in 2017, and 9.53 million stroke survivors, 0.46 million deaths and 7.06 million lost disability-adjusted life years (DALYs) were counted [31]. Globally, there is one stroke each three seconds and one in four people will suffer from stroke during their lifetime [16]. Moreover, incidence and prevalence are expected to rise in the future, due to aging of the population. Two types with different origin can be discriminated: ischemic stroke caused by a blood clot (a thrombosis or an embolism), and hemorrhagic stroke caused by bleeding. In Europe, 80% of strokes is ischemic, while in the USA, ischemic stroke accounts for even 87% of all cases [5,30].

Because it is often difficult to discriminate ischemic from hemorrhagic stroke based on the patient's symptoms, neuroimaging techniques such as computed tomography (CT) or magnetic resonance imaging (MRI) are required. In the acute setting, CT is often preferred for the diagnosis of stroke in most hospitals, because of its fast acquisition, accessibility, and availability [24]. A non-contrast enhanced CT scan (NCCT) can be used to discriminate between both types, but more specific stroke characteristics such as cerebral blood flow and cerebral blood volume, which give a general idea about the lesion volume, severity, and possible benefits of treatment, are obtained and evaluated with CT perfusion imaging (CTP).

For ischemic stroke, there are two acute treatment options, aiming at restoring the normal perfusion of the brain by recanalization: intravenous injection of a thrombolytic drug, such as recombinant tissue plasminogen activator (rtPA), and, in case of large vessel occlusion (LVO), endovascular treatment (EVT) where the clot is mechanically removed. LVO strokes account for 24% to 46% of all acute ischemic strokes (AIS) [22]. Both treatments have a specific time window after the onset of stroke which is longer for EVT in comparison to rtPA.

The final goal of stroke treatment is to improve the functional outcome of patients thereby achieving a good quality of life. The functional outcome is often defined in terms of the modified Rankin Scale (mRS) score, three months after stroke onset. This scoring system measures the degree of disability/dependence in the daily activities of patients who suffered from a stroke, ranging from no residual symptoms (mRS = 0) to dead (mRS = 6). The mRS score is often binarized in favorable outcome (mRS 0-2) versus unfavorable outcome (mRS 3-6). Research has indicated several relevant variables which influence functional outcome. First, patient-specific factors have been identified, such as age, sex, prior medical treatments, recurrent stroke, and collateral circulation (i.e., a supplementary vessel circuit along which an additional supply of blood flow is possible) [2,8,15,27,32]. Second, also stroke severity plays a role, which is often assessed with the National Institutes of Health Stroke Scale (NIHSS) at admission and 24 h after stroke onset [26]. Third, treatment parameters such as time from stroke onset to EVT and modified Thrombolysis in Cerebral Infarction (mTICI) score after reperfusion (which evaluates the extent of reperfusion after EVT using a scale from grade 0 to 3) have also been shown to affect functional outcome [14,21,34]. Lastly, using techniques such as voxel-based lesion-symptom mapping (VLSM), the relationship between neurological deficits and the corresponding lesion location in the brain is shown [4,12]. In current literature, final infarct volume and lesion location are often assessed together by using lesion loads of each anatomical region. This predictive biomarker is the percentage of volume of the region that is affected by the lesion [17].

Reliable functional outcome prediction models that incorporate treatment variables as input, could be used to guide the medical staff assessing the benefit-risk balance of different treatment options, allowing to select an optimal treatment strategy tailored to the individual patient. Moreover, the medical team could anticipate on a predicted poor patient outcome. Also, it would allow for an optimal planning of discharge, rehabilitation, and end-of-life care.

Recently, artificial intelligence (AI)-based approaches using conventional machine learning (ML) models, such as logistic regression, support vector machines, decision tree-based models and multilayer perceptrons, have been studied for functional outcome prediction [1,19,29]. ML models are flexible in terms of input features, allowing them to exploit a broad range of input variables going from patient data (e.g., age, sex, clinical history) to radiological biomarkers (e.g., presence of intracranial atherosclerosis and/or old infarcts). Moreover, they allow to easily simulate the effect of individual input variables (e.g., different treatment options) on the predicted outcome. ML models have been shown to outperform conventional scores such as the Alberta Stroke Program Early CT Score (ASPECTS) [3] for the prediction of mRS six months after stroke onset [19]. Nevertheless, the potential of current such models for outcome prediction in stroke is often still limited by using either clinical data (e.g., age, sex) or imaging data (e.g., radiological biomarkers) but not both. However, recent research has reported a positive effect on model performance of combining different types of input variables, such as imaging data with clinical data [25,28]. Furthermore, treatment parameters (such as EVT performed or not, time to EVT) are only seldomly included in these models. Another limitation of current outcome prediction models is their lack of applicability and clinical benefit in the acute setting. This is mainly because they rely on input parameters collected during follow-up, such as NIHSS at 24 h after stroke onset, which has been shown to improve performance but prevents application of the prediction model during the acute treatment phase [10].

We hypothesize a beneficial effect of adding treatment parameters to acutely available clinical variables for the prediction of functional outcome of AIS patients treated with EVT. Also, we hypothesize the additional information provided by the treatment variables being indirectly present in the follow-up NCCT scan.

2 Methods

2.1 Data Set

Two distinctive data sets were used, containing patients with AIS in the anterior circulation caused by a LVO. Both data sets consist of imaging data (acute CTP, acute NCCT and follow-up NCCT) as well as clinical and treatment variables (age, sex, NIHSS score at admission, rtPA administration, mTICI score after EVT, time from stroke onset to EVT and mRS score three months after stroke onset among others).

The first data set was derived from a randomized clinical trial from the Netherlands (MR CLEAN) [6]. The derived cohort contained patients with the presence of a CTP and follow-up NCCT of sufficient quality, resulting in 188 cases. Patients not treated with EVT (n=100) were excluded. Of the remaining cohort, patients with an insufficient axial field of view of the CTP were discarded (n=41), such that exactly the same patients can be used in future research projects involving CTP. Eventually, this resulted in a total of 47 cases. As ground truth, the delineations of the core lesion on follow-up NCCT of [11] were used.

The second data set was derived from an in-house data set of AIS patients admitted to the Karolinska University Hospital in Stockholm (Sweden), containing patients all treated with EVT [7]. After excluding cases with CT scans of insufficient quality, 385 cases were retained. The final core lesions were delineated on follow-up NCCT. 1/3 was delineated by a neuroradiologist, 1/3 by a neurologist and 1/3 by both raters separately. Cases where the necessary metadata (age, sex, NIHSS score at admission, rtPA administration, mTICI score after EVT, time from stroke onset to EVT and mRS score three months after stroke onset) were not available (n = 171) were excluded, leading eventually to 214 patients.

Together, the two data sets generated one large data set of 261 patients with imaging of sufficient quality and other metadata in the form of clinical and treatment variables.

2.2 Input Features

Three types of input features were used for training of the models. First, clinical data available in the acute phase: age, sex and NIHSS score at admission. Second, treatment variables: rtPA administration, mTICI score after EVT, time from stroke onset to EVT. Third, imaging data: lesion loads. To assess the lesion loads of the patients, follow-up NCCT scans made 24 h after stroke onset were registered to a stroke population-specific neuroanatomical CT brain atlas [18]. This atlas contains 116 anatomical brain regions and was specifically created for stroke research. It is based on images of 50 subjects that are age and sex matched to a typical stroke population, with a median age of 71.9 years and of whom 60% were males. The NCCT scans were registered in three steps: a translation, an affine transformation and a non-rigid transformation. Both the translation and affine transformation were executed using mutual information. For the non-rigid transformation, normalized cross-correlation was used. The registration algorithm was implemented in Python using *SimpleElastix* [20]. Cases where the registration failed were excluded, resulting in a final data set of 236 patients, of whom 116 (49%) had a favorable outcome (mRS 0-2) three months after stroke onset and 120 (51%) had an unfavorable outcome (mRS 3-6). 124 patients (53%) were male and 112 (47%) female. The mean age was 68 years (minimum: 28 years, maximum: 90 years). The mean time from stroke onset to EVT was 5 h and 43 min (minimum: 1 h and 32 min, maximum: 20 h and 11 min).

Of the 116 regions in the Kaffenberger atlas, some regions are drained by the posterior circulation, and some are not or little affected by the strokes present in the data set. Therefore, regions with an average lesion load per case smaller than 1% were excluded from the set of input features. Also, all clinical and treatment variables were scaled with respect to a fixed value (for age: 100 years, for scores such as NIHSS: maximum score, for time-related values: 24 h). Principal Component Analysis (PCA) was performed on the lesion loads of the training cases. The number of principal components was selected based on a cumulative variance of 95%, resulting in 21 or 22 components (depending on the training fold). The final principal component values were scaled with respect to the maximum value of that component over all training cases. The same PCA transformation and scaling of the training set was applied on the test case, defined by a leave-one-out cross-validation (LOOCV) strategy.

2.3 Models

To asses the effect of input variables on model performance, an ensemble model consisting of five ML models was trained: 1) logistic regression (LR) (solver = limited-memory Broyden-Fletcher-Goldfarb-Shanno), 2) support vector machine (SVM) (kernel = polynomial), 3) random forest (RF) (number of trees = 200, split criterion = Gini impurity), 4) multilayer perceptron (MLP) (number of hidden layers = 3, neurons per hidden layer = 10), 5) k-nearest neighbors (KNN) (number of neighbors = 9). The models were individually trained on the training data to predict favorable versus unfavorable outcome and applied on the test case using a LOOCV strategy to extract probability predictions. Platt scaling was used to convert the binary class prediction of the SVM model to a probability prediction. Likewise, for the RF model, a probability prediction was calculated by dividing the number of votes of the trees by the number of trees in the forest. A similar strategy was applied in case of the KNN model, where the votes of the neighbors were divided by the number of neighbors. The probability predictions of the five individual ML models were averaged to obtain one prediction of the ensemble model, where each individual ML model prediction contributed equally to the final ensemble average probability (uniform weighting). Afterwards, the ensemble probability was dichotomized in favorable and unfavorable outcome using a threshold of $\geq$0.5. The performance of the ensemble model was evaluated using the predictions of all folds. The model's accuracy,

AUC, sensitivity, specificity and F1-score was assessed, with unfavorable outcome indicated as the positive class. The training and validation algorithm of the models was implemented in Python using *Scikit-Learn* and *Keras* [13,23]. Statistical significance of the accuracy scores was tested using a two-sided Wilcoxon signed-rank test, with a p-value of 0.05.

3 Results

The performance metrics of the ensemble model and the individual ML models are displayed in Table 1. A distinction is made between the used input features (clinical variables, lesion loads and/or treatment variables). For the set of input features consisting of clinical variables, treatment variables and lesion loads, the difference in performance between the ensemble model and the LR, RF and MLP models was found to be statistically significant. Also when using clinical variables and lesion loads as input features, the difference in performance between the ensemble model and the LR, RF and MLP models was shown to be statistically significant. When clinical and treatment variables were used as input features, or when only clinical variables were used, no statistically significant difference was found between the results of the ensemble model and the individual ML models.

Comparing only the ensemble models, no statistically significant difference in performance between two distinct sets of input features was found.

4 Discussion

From the six models (five individual ML models and one ensemble model), the ensemble model and SVM seem to perform best over all possible sets of input features (Table 1), taking into account five performance metrics (accuracy, AUC, sensitivity, specificity and F1-score). The obtained performances are in line with other research [35].

Remarkably, little variance in the performance metrics is found across the different sets of input features. Possibly, the applied ML models are too simplistic to capture the complex interactions between the various variables. More sophisticated models such as deep learning models might be necessary to obtain robust and reliable classification algorithms with better performance. Furthermore, the similar performances across the different sets of input features might be (partially) explained by high variability in the input and target data, due to the various intermediate steps of the pipeline. Inconsistency in the data could be present because of inter-rater variability of the mRS score [33,36], inter-rater variability of the delineations [9], variability in the measurement of the time from stroke onset to treatment, variability due to the registration algorithm, limited resolution of the neuroanatomical CT brain atlas, etc. This could result in patterns which are divergent over the various training samples and hamper model convergence.

The effect of adding treatment parameters to a model using clinical features and lesion loads is expected to be minimal, as the lesion loads are derived from

Table 1. Performance metrics of the individual machine learning models (LR = logistic regression, SVM = support vector machine, RF = random forest, MLP = multilayer perceptron, KNN = k-nearest neighbors). C = clinical features, L = lesion loads, T = treatment parameters. Per set of input features and per performance metric, the highest performance value is indicated in bold.

Input features	Model	Accuracy	AUC	Sensitivity	Specificity	F1-score
C + L + T	Ensemble	0.68	0.70	0.67	0.69	0.68
	LR	0.64	0.71	0.46	**0.84**	0.57
	SVM	**0.69**	0.71	0.67	0.72	0.69
	RF	0.59	**0.74**	**0.97**	0.20	**0.71**
	MLP	0.53	0.60	0.78	0.28	0.63
	KNN	0.65	0.69	0.70	0.60	0.67
C + L	Ensemble	**0.68**	0.74	0.69	0.66	0.69
	LR	0.64	0.71	0.45	**0.84**	0.56
	SVM	0.67	0.71	0.71	0.63	0.69
	RF	0.61	**0.75**	**0.96**	0.24	**0.71**
	MLP	0.58	0.62	0.87	0.28	0.68
	KNN	**0.68**	0.71	0.76	0.59	**0.71**
C + T	Ensemble	0.69	0.76	0.72	0.67	0.70
	LR	0.69	0.74	0.70	0.69	0.70
	SVM	**0.72**	**0.77**	0.72	**0.73**	**0.73**
	RF	0.70	0.76	0.73	0.67	0.71
	MLP	0.59	0.59	**0.81**	0.36	0.67
	KNN	0.65	0.66	0.64	0.66	0.65
C	Ensemble	0.69	0.73	0.72	0.66	0.70
	LR	0.69	0.73	0.69	0.69	0.69
	SVM	**0.70**	**0.76**	0.70	**0.70**	0.70
	RF	0.67	0.73	0.69	0.65	0.69
	MLP	0.64	0.70	0.68	0.61	0.66
	KNN	**0.70**	0.70	**0.75**	0.65	**0.72**

the follow-up NCCT scan, which is assumed to contain the final core lesion which does not expand anymore. Indeed, no statistically significant difference was found between the ensemble model using clinical variables, treatment variables and lesion loads and the ensemble model using only clinical variables and lesion loads. In contrast, in a model using only clinical variables, adding treatment parameters as input features could possibly improve the model's performance. However, this expected pattern is not visible in the results depicted in Table 1, possibly due to the aforementioned reasons concerning complexity of the models and variability in the intermediate steps of the pipeline.

Nevertheless, all sets of input variables include clinical variables. Together with the low variance of the performance metrics, this suggest the importance of basic clinical variables (age, sex and NIHSS at admission) in functional outcome prediction models. These variables are mostly available in an acute stroke setting, which makes them ideal candidates for future outcome prediction models.

5 Conclusion

Functional outcome prediction models are desirable to improve stroke health care. Out of six ML models, the SVM model and an ensemble model seem to perform best. Although ML models achieve moderate performances, the complex interactions between variables might require more sophisticated models to obtain robust and reliable prediction models.

References

1. Alaka, S.A., et al.: Functional outcome prediction in ischemic stroke: a comparison of machine learning algorithms and regression models. Front. Neurol. **11**, 889 (2020). https://doi.org/10.3389/fneur.2020.00889
2. Bang, O.Y., Goyal, M., Liebeskind, D.S.: Collateral circulation in ischemic stroke: assessment tools and therapeutic strategies. Stroke **46**(11), 3302–3309 (2015). https://doi.org/10.1161/STROKEAHA.115.010508
3. Barber, P.A., Demchuk, A.M., Zhang, J., Buchan, A.M.: Validity and reliability of a quantitative computed tomography score in predicting outcome of hyperacute stroke before thrombolytic therapy. Lancet **355**(9216), 1670–1674 (2000). https://doi.org/10.1016/s0140-6736(00)02237-6
4. Bates, E., et al.: Voxel-based lesion-symptom mapping. Nat. Neurosci. **6**(5), 448–450 (2003). https://doi.org/10.1038/nn1050
5. Béjot, Y., Bailly, H., Durier, J., Giroud, M.: Epidemiology of stroke in Europe and trends for the 21st century. La Presse Médicale **45**(12), e391–e398 (2016). https://doi.org/10.1016/j.lpm.2016.10.003
6. Berkhemer, O.A., et al.: A randomized trial of intraarterial treatment for acute ischemic stroke. NEJM **372**, 11–20 (2015). https://doi.org/10.1056/NEJMoa1411587
7. Bertels, J.: Understanding final infarct prediction in acute ischemic stroke using convolutional neural networks. Ph.D. thesis, KU Leuven (2022). https://lirias.kuleuven.be/3838597?limo=0
8. Black-Schaffer, R.M., Winston, C.: Age and functional outcome after stroke. Top. Stroke Rehabil. **11**(2), 23–32 (2004). https://doi.org/10.1310/DNJU-9VUH-BXU2-DJYU
9. Boers, A.M., et al.: Automated cerebral infarct volume measurement in follow-up noncontrast CT scans of patients with acute ischemic stroke. Am. J. Neuroradiol. **34**(8), 1522–1527 (2013). https://doi.org/10.3174/ajnr.A3463
10. Brugnara, G., et al.: Multimodal predictive modeling of endovascular treatment outcome for acute ischemic stroke using machine-learning. Stroke **51**(12), 3541–3551 (2020). https://doi.org/10.1161/STROKEAHA.120.030287

11. Bucker, A., et al.: Associations of ischemic lesion volume with functional outcome in patients with acute ischemic stroke: 24-hour versus 1-week imaging. Stroke **48**(5), 1233–1240 (2017). https://doi.org/10.1161/STROKEAHA.116.015156
12. Cheng, B., et al.: Influence of stroke infarct location on functional outcome measured by the modified Rankin Scale. Stroke **45**(6), 1695–1702 (2014). https://doi.org/10.1161/STROKEAHA.114.005152
13. Chollet, F., et al.: Keras (2015). https://keras.io. Accessed 20 June 2023
14. Dargazanli, C., et al.: Impact of modified TICI 3 versus modified TICI 2b reperfusion score to predict good outcome following endovascular therapy. Am. J. Neuroradiol. **38**(1), 90–96 (2017). https://doi.org/10.3174/ajnr.A4968
15. Demeestere, J., et al.: Effect of sex on clinical outcome and imaging after endovascular treatment of large-vessel ischemic stroke. J. Stroke Cerebrovasc. Dis. **30**(2), 105468 (2021). https://doi.org/10.1016/j.jstrokecerebrovasdis.2020.105468
16. Feigin, V.L., et al.: World stroke organization (WSO): global stroke fact sheet 2022. Int. J. Stroke **17**(1), 18–29 (2022). https://doi.org/10.1177/17474930211065917
17. Habegger, S., et al.: Relating acute lesion loads to chronic outcome in ischemic stroke-an exploratory comparison of mismatch patterns and predictive modeling. Front. Neurol. **9**, 737 (2018). https://doi.org/10.3389/fneur.2018.00737
18. Kaffenberger, T., et al.: Stroke population-specific neuroanatomical CT-MRI brain atlas. Neuroradiology **64**(8), 1557–1567 (2022). https://doi.org/10.1007/s00234-021-02875-9
19. Li, X., et al.: Predicting 6-month unfavorable outcome of acute ischemic stroke using machine learning. Front. Neurol. **11**, 539509 (2020). https://doi.org/10.3389/fneur.2020.539509
20. Marstal, K., Berendsen, F., Staring, M., Klein, S.: SimplEelastix: a user-friendly, multi-lingual library for medical image registration. In: Proceedings of the IEEE Conference on Computer Vision and Pattern Recognition Workshops, pp. 134–142 (2016). https://doi.org/10.1109/CVPRW.2016.78
21. Mazighi, M., et al.: Impact of onset-to-reperfusion time on stroke mortality: a collaborative pooled analysis. Circulation **127**(19), 1980–1985 (2013). https://doi.org/10.1161/CIRCULATIONAHA.112.000311
22. Nicholls, J.K., Ince, J., Minhas, J.S., Chung, E.M.: Emerging detection techniques for large vessel occlusion stroke: a scoping review. Front. Neurol. **12**, 2477 (2022). https://doi.org/10.3389/fneur.2021.780324
23. Pedregosa, F., et al.: Scikit-learn: machine learning in python. J. Mach. Learn. Res. **12**, 2825–2830 (2011). https://www.jmlr.org/papers/v12/pedregosa11a.html
24. Phipps, M.S., Cronin, C.A.: Management of acute ischemic stroke. BMJ **368** (2020). https://doi.org/10.1136/bmj.l6983
25. Ramos, L.A., et al.: Combination of radiological and clinical baseline data for outcome prediction of patients with an acute ischemic stroke. Front. Neurol., 602 (2022). https://doi.org/10.3389/fneur.2022.809343
26. Reznik, M.E., et al.: Baseline NIH stroke scale is an inferior predictor of functional outcome in the era of acute stroke intervention. Int. J. Stroke **13**(8), 806–810 (2018). https://doi.org/10.1177/1747493018783759
27. Sacco, S., Toni, D., Bignamini, A.A., Zaninelli, A., Gensini, G.F.: Effect of prior medical treatments on ischemic stroke severity and outcome. Funct. Neurol. **26**(3), 133 (2011). https://www.ncbi.nlm.nih.gov/pmc/articles/PMC3814556/
28. Tolhuisen, M.L., et al.: Outcome prediction based on automatically extracted infarct core image features in patients with acute ischemic stroke. Diagnostics **12**(8), 1786 (2022). https://doi.org/10.3390/diagnostics12081786

29. Van Os, H.J., et al.: Predicting outcome of endovascular treatment for acute ischemic stroke: potential value of machine learning algorithms. Front. Neurol. **9**, 784 (2018). https://doi.org/10.3389/fneur.2018.00784
30. Virani, S.S., et al.: Heart disease and stroke statistics-2020 update: a report from the American heart association. Circulation **141**(9), e139–e596 (2020). https://doi.org/10.1161/CIR.0000000000000757
31. Wafa, H.A., Wolfe, C.D., Emmett, E., Roth, G.A., Johnson, C.O., Wang, Y.: Burden of stroke in Europe: thirty-year projections of incidence, prevalence, deaths, and disability-adjusted life years. Stroke **51**(8), 2418–2427 (2020). https://doi.org/10.1161/STROKEAHA.120.029606
32. Wang, A., et al.: Effect of recurrent stroke on poor functional outcome in transient ischemic attack or minor stroke. Int. J. Stroke **11**(7), NP80 (2016). https://doi.org/10.1177/1747493016641954
33. Wilson, J.L., Hareendran, A., Hendry, A., Potter, J., Bone, I., Muir, K.W.: Reliability of the modified Rankin Scale across multiple raters: benefits of a structured interview. Stroke **36**(4), 777–781 (2005). https://doi.org/10.1161/01.STR.0000157596.13234.95
34. Zaidat, O.O., et al.: Recommendations on angiographic revascularization grading standards for acute ischemic stroke: a consensus statement. Stroke **44**(9), 2650–2663 (2013). https://doi.org/10.1161/STROKEAHA.113.001972
35. Zeng, M., et al.: Pre-thrombectomy prognostic prediction of large-vessel ischemic stroke using machine learning: a systematic review and meta-analysis. Front. Neurol. **13**, 945813 (2022). https://doi.org/10.3389/fneur.2022.945813
36. Zhao, H., Collier, J.M., Quah, D.M., Purvis, T., Bernhardt, J.: The modified Rankin Scale in acute stroke has good inter-rater-reliability but questionable validity. Cerebrovasc. Dis. **29**(2), 188–193 (2010). https://doi.org/10.1159/000267278

The Detection and Segmentation of Blush in the Lenticulostriate Territory

Sjir J. C. Schielen[1](✉), Danny H. Huynh[1], Bart A. J. M. Wagemans[2], Danny Ruijters[1], Wim H. van Zwam[2], and Svitlana Zinger[1]

[1] Eindhoven University of Technology, Eindhoven, The Netherlands
s.j.c.schielen@tue.nl

[2] Department of Radiology and Nuclear Medicine, Maastricht University Medical Center, Maastricht, The Netherlands

Abstract. The lenticulostriate territory is a region in the brain that is only supplied by lenticulostriate vessels. As this region does not benefit from collateral blood flow, it warrants attention in the event of ischemic stroke. Perfusion in the lenticulostriate territory shows up as a blush in digital subtraction angiography. Although this blush is observable, visual inspection is subjective and qualitative while a quantitative figure of merit is desired. To allow quantitative analysis of this blush, a segmentation of the correct blush is necessary. In this paper, a deep-learning approach is proposed to perform the novel segmentation of the blush in the lenticulostriate territory. To provide a first quantification of the blush, the hemisphere in which it occurred is also segmented. The ratio between these segmentations is a quantification of the size of the blush compared to the size of the hemisphere. Results indicate proof of concept, but more steps are needed before clinical application.

Keywords: Deep Learning · Segmentation · Lenticulostriate Vessels · Stroke · Blush

1 Introduction

Ischemic stroke occurs when an artery in the brain is blocked, preventing it from supplying blood to successive vessels and tissues. Stroke is the second leading cause of death worldwide [9]. Endovascular treatments, such as thrombectomy, are effective clinical treatments for ischemic stroke when added to usual care [7].

Endovascular treatments are executed under guidance of medical-imaging technologies such as interventional X-ray. To visualize the vessels of interest in X-ray imaging, digital subtraction angiography (DSA) is performed [6]. DSA is a technique where a mask image is made prior to the injection of contrast fluid. The mask image is then digitally subtracted from subsequent images, allowing a clearer visualization of vascular structures and blushes of contrast fluid.

Perforating vessels that branch from e.g. the arteria cerebri media supply blood to a specific region of the brain named the lenticulostriate territory [2].

U. Baid et al. (Eds.): BrainLes 2023/SWITCH 2023, LNCS 14668, pp. 134–143, 2024.
https://doi.org/10.1007/978-3-031-76160-7_13

Whereas other regions of the brain may be supplied by collateral blood flow besides their primary source, the lenticulostriate territory is not supplied with collateral blood flow. Therefore, the perforating vessels, or lenticulostriate vessels, are this region's main and only source of blood.

Given the importance of lenticulostriate vessels to the survival of the tissues forming the lenticulostriate territory, the perfusion in this region warrants attention in the event of lenticulostriate infarction or occlusion of preceding vessels. Perfusion occurs at the cellular level and the lenticulostriate capillaries' width can range from 100 μm to 400 μm [11]. As DSA, like any imaging technique, is limited in its spatial resolution, the smaller vessels and perfusion are not visualized as clear structures but rather as a blush. An example of a blush in the lenticulostriate territory is shown in Fig. 1. Valuable information is contained in whether a blush is visible and, if it is visible, how much. Visual examination of these blushes is subjective and qualitative, where ultimately a quantitative measurement is desired. Therefore, the idea is proposed to automate the detection of blush in the lenticulostriate territory.

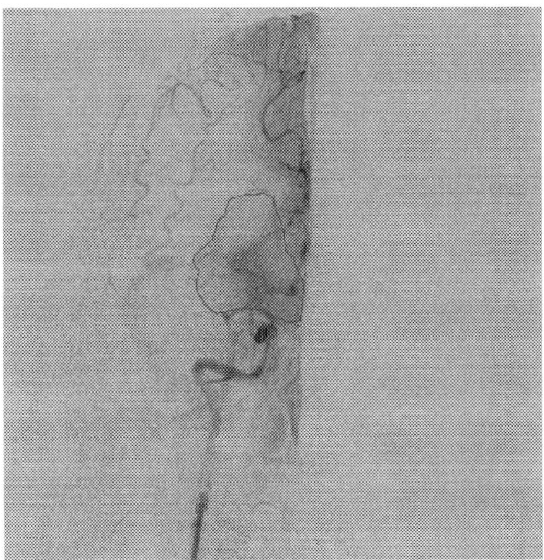

Fig. 1. Digital subtraction angiography where a somewhat visible blush in the lenticulostriate territory is contoured with blue (Color figure online).

While studies have focused on a description or quantification of the physical morphometry of the visible lenticulostriate arteries using magnetic resonance imaging [16,17], no investigations of the smaller vessels or blush in the lenticulostriate territory seem to exist. No directly applicable studies were found after an honest research attempt, therefore related work with some overlap is considered.

Deep-learning-based detection in DSA is used for intracranial aneurysms [10] and vessel punctures during an intervention [12] with satisfactory results. In these applications, however, the distinction between the background and the region of interest (ROI) seems clearer than the distinction between blush and the background may be in DSA. This vaguer distinction between the ROI and the background can also be observed in computed tomography (CT) imaging of intracranial hemorrhage. Convolutional neural networks are applied to classify intracranial hemorrhages [1,3] and to the bounding-box segmentation of these hemorrhages [3]. Both the former and the latter applications are performed on CT instead of interventional X-ray images. Although the results are promising, there are discrepancies between intracranial hemorrhages in CT and the blush in the lenticulostriate territory in DSA.

Promising related work shows potential in the application of deep-learning-based methods for blush detection in the lenticulostriate territory. Therefore, the aim of this paper is to apply deep learning to segment the blush in the lenticulostriate territory. Two main contributions are made. To the best of our knowledge, this is the first segmentation of blush in the lenticulostriate territory. Furthermore, the obtained segmentations serve as input for quantitative analysis. This is exemplified by calculating the ratio between the blush in the lenticulostriate territory and the segmentation of the hemisphere. Such quantification may be used to investigate treatment effectivity and prognosis.

In the remainder of this paper, the methodology is presented first. Then, the results following from this methodology are reported and discussed and finally, conclusions are drawn.

2 Methodology

The step-by-step approach is shown in Fig. 2. The system takes a frame of a DSA-image array without any annotations as input and yields a version that contains a bounding box around the blush in the lenticulostriate territory. The steps of the approach are described separately in this section.

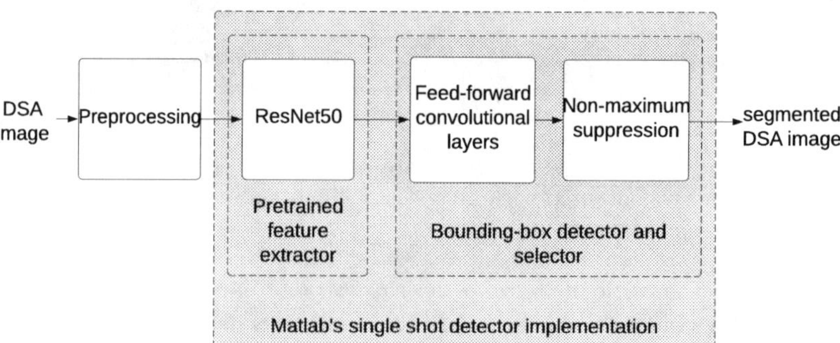

Fig. 2. A flowchart of the proposed methodology. DSA - digital subtraction angiography, ResNet - residual network (Color figure online)

2.1 Preprocessing

The difference between related ROI detections (e.g. an aneurysm or vessel puncture [10,12]) and the detection of blush in the lenticulostriate territory is the distinction between the ROI and the background. Blush may be present in low intensity, not resulting in a clearly defined border between blush and background. Therefore, contrast enhancement is applied using Matlab's `imadjust` function that saturates the top and bottom 1% of the grayscale pixel values [13]. An example is shown in Fig. 3a.

While the blush in the lenticulostriate territory deviates in shape from a rectangle, still the decision is made to use bounding-box segmentations. As it may be challenging to differentiate between the blush and the background, the risk of missing part of the blush is lower with a wider outline. Exact delineations are more time-consuming as a consensus of different experts is required. Moreover, noise and motion artifacts may degrade image quality making exact delineations more difficult. If a bounding-box segmentation is placed correctly over the blush but a little wider than strictly necessary, the required information can still be used in postprocessing. Therefore, the interest in the correct general placement of the bounding box is preferred over the exact delineation of the blush.

Data augmentation in the form of mirroring and moderate rotations is applied to enlarge the training set. Rotations are limited between 3° and 10° to not introduce features considered unrealistic. An example of a rotated image is shown in Fig. 3b. The bounding boxes are manually created for both the blush in the lenticulostriate and the brain hemisphere in which the blush occurs. These segmentations are aided by input from clinicians. A bounding-box segmentation of the blush is shown in Fig. 3c and a bounding box around the hemisphere is shown in Fig. 3d.

2.2 Single Shot Detector

The used deep-learning architecture is highlighted in green in Fig. 2, which follows Matlab's implementation [14] of the Single Shot Detector (SSD) architecture [8]. The first part is a pretrained feature extractor which is shown in blue in Fig. 2. In this implementation, the first 40 layers of the 50-layer residual network (ResNet) [5] serve as the feature extractor. The feature extractor is pretrained on a vehicle dataset [15]. A pretrained model gives the benefit of familiarity with high-level features that can be tailored to new use cases. This is particularly useful in applications with small datasets, which often is the case in medical applications.

The next part (red in Fig. 2) detects and selects bounding boxes from the extracted features. Convolutional layers that progressively decrease in size are cascaded. The output of each layer is fed to both the next layer and forward to the non-maximum suppression part. This results in many potential bounding boxes. Non-maximum suppression uses Jaccard overlap to discard most of the found bounding boxes [8]. The output of the feature extractor is also used for classification. Only classified objects receive a bounding box in the final image.

The loss function is a combination of a term that aims to get the bounding box in the correct place and a term that checks the correct classification of the object in the box. The localization loss of the bounding box $\mathcal{L}_{loc}(x, l, g)$ is computed by

$$\mathcal{L}_{loc}(x, l, g) = \sum_{i \in Pos}^{N} \sum_{m \in bp} x_i \text{smooth}_{L_1}(l_i^m - \hat{g}_j^m), \tag{1}$$

where x_i is a binary indicator for the matching of the i-th bounding box in the set of possible bounding boxes Pos with cardinality N. Furthermore, the parameters l and g represent respectively the predicted and the ground-truth box. The term smooth_{L_1} is a smoother version of the L_1-norm given by

$$\text{smooth}_{L_1}(x) = \begin{cases} 0.5x^2, & \text{if } |x| < 1 \\ |x| - 0.5, & \text{otherwise,} \end{cases} \tag{2}$$

which is introduced in [4]. The set bp used in the second summation of (1) refers to the bounding-box parameters, i.e. the way a box is numerically represented. A box is represented as corner coordinates (cx, cy), a width w, and a height h: $bp = \{cx, cy, w, h\}$. Note that in 1 $\hat{g}$ is used as the argument of smooth_{L_1} instead of g. This indicates that the predicted bounding-box parameters are compared to the ground-truth bounding-box parameters differently per parameter. The full mathematical derivation is provided in [8].

The loss term used for classification is binary cross entropy $\mathcal{L}_{BCE}$:

$$\mathcal{L}_{BCE}(y, p) = -\sum y \log(p) + (1 - y) \log(1 - p), \tag{3}$$

where y if the ground-truth label and p is the predicted probability of the label. This results in the total loss function $\mathcal{L}$:

$$\mathcal{L} = \mathcal{L}_{loc}(x, l, g) + \mathcal{L}_{BCE}(y, p). \tag{4}$$

The architecture is designed to both localize an object and check if it is present in the first place. This can be directly applied to blush as it may not be present either because of the absence of perfusion or because the contrast fluid has not reached it yet. The localization part is needed because blush may show up outside of the lenticulostriate territory (e.g. at the top of Fig. 3a), but specifically the blush in the lenticulostriate territory is of interest. This approach also works for the segmentation of the hemisphere as it should be present but the contrast fluid may not have reached it yet to make it visible.

2.3 Evaluation

To evaluate the performance of the network, two different metrics are used. The first metric is the mean intersection over union $mIoU$:

$$mIoU = \frac{1}{N} \sum_{i}^{N} \frac{g_i \cap l_i}{g_i \cup l_i}, \tag{5}$$

where N indicates the size of the test set. Note that a slight abuse of notation is introduced by reusing N after equation (1), but generally it is used to describe the size of the set, vector, etc. The second metric is the mean Sørensen-Dice index $mSDI$, which is given by

$$mSDI = \frac{1}{N}\sum_{i}^{N} 2\frac{g_i \cap l_i}{g_i + l_i}. \tag{6}$$

These metrics are for bounding-box segmentations. An example quantitative score for the size of the blush is the ratio between the size of the bounding box of the blush and the size of the bounding box of the hemisphere. This ratio can be computed between ground-truth boxes and predicted boxes and the mean squared error (MSE) between them is computed. For example, the ratio between blush (Fig. 3c) and hemisphere (Fig. 3d) is 0.24, meaning that lenticulostriate blush accounts for about a quarter of the hemisphere.

3 Results

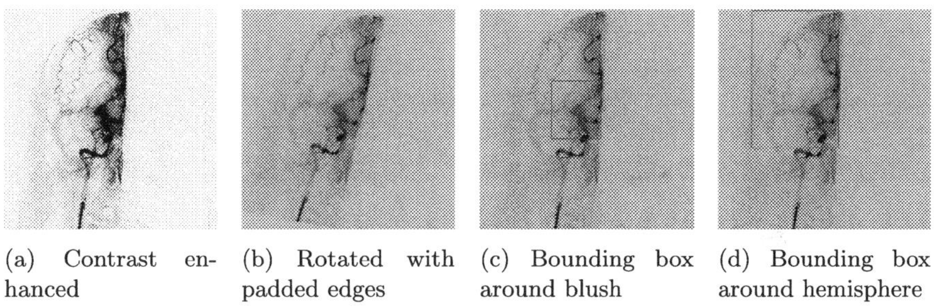

(a) Contrast enhanced (b) Rotated with padded edges (c) Bounding box around blush (d) Bounding box around hemisphere

Fig. 3. Examples of augmentations and bounding boxes

3.1 Dataset

A dataset was acquired at Maastricht University Medical Center (MUMC) with permission of MUMC's medical ethics committee. Patients were sought that had an acute ischemic stroke and underwent mechanical thrombectomy. If patients had a recurrent stroke, only the first stroke was included in the dataset, hence the dataset exists of unique patients. Arrays of DSA images taken in anteroposterior view were retrieved. The motivation for the anteroposterior view is that the lenticulostriate territory can be more easily identified than in other views. Patients were excluded if the viewpoint deviated too much from anteroposterior, if the basilar artery syndrome was present, or if motion artifacts severely degraded image quality.

As only the images themselves are of interest for the development of an algorithm, additional information (e.g. demographics) was anonymized. A total of 100 patients were included in the dataset, of which 73 had a visible blush in the lenticulostriate territory. In total 316 unique frames with a visible blush were available for model training, validation, and testing.

While transfer learning compensates partly for the size limitation of the dataset, the augmentation described in the methods section (2.1) is applied to increase the combined size of the training and validation set by approximately 30%. Data augmentation is exclusively used on training and validation sets to ensure that test results represent performance on clinical inputs. In this way, training and testing on information originating from the same patient is also avoided. Patients are randomly subdivided over the train (51), validation (10), and test set (12). Before augmentation, the number of frames in each set is 218, 47, and 51 respectively. After augmentation, the number of frames in the training and validation set is increased to 283 and 61 respectively.

3.2 Evaluation

Table 1. The obtained results for the predefined evaluation metrics: $mIoU$ - mean intersection over union, $mSDI$ - mean Sørensen-Dice index

	no enhancement		enhanced	
	$mIoU$	$mSDI$	$mIoU$	$mSDI$
Blush	0.461	0.598	0.498	0.634
Hemisphere	0.736	0.838	0.734	0.835

The evaluation metrics computed on the predicted bounding-box placements of the test set are listed in Table 1. Furthermore, as an example of a quantification of blush in the lenticulostriate territory, the ratio between the bounding box around the blush and the bounding box around the hemisphere is computed for both the predicted bounding boxes and the ground-truth bounding boxes. The mean squared error between the output and ground-truth ratios is computed, which resulted in 0.0088 without contrast enhancement and 0.0051 with contrast enhancement. The root can be taken which results in respectively 0.09 and 0.07, which means an average error of 9% and 7%.

To give some interpretation to the results, the metrics $mIoU$ and $mSDI$ are both limited between 0 and 1 and indicate the degree of overlap between the predicted and ground-truth bounding boxes. As can be seen in Table 1, the blush is harder to predict than the hemisphere, which is partly due to the difference in size between the blush and hemisphere. Also, the distinction between the ROI and the background is clearer for the hemisphere than for the blush.

It is visible that contrast enhancement improves performance for the segmentation of the blush (Table 1). This is in line with the a-priori expectation that the vaguer distinction between the blush and the background contributes most to the difficulty of this segmentation problem. This can be further supported by observing the results of the segmentation of the hemisphere, where the enhancement does not make a clear difference.

Overall, the results for the segmentation of the blush can be considered moderately well (with contrast enhancement) and for the segmentation of the hemisphere the results are good (independent of contrast enhancement).

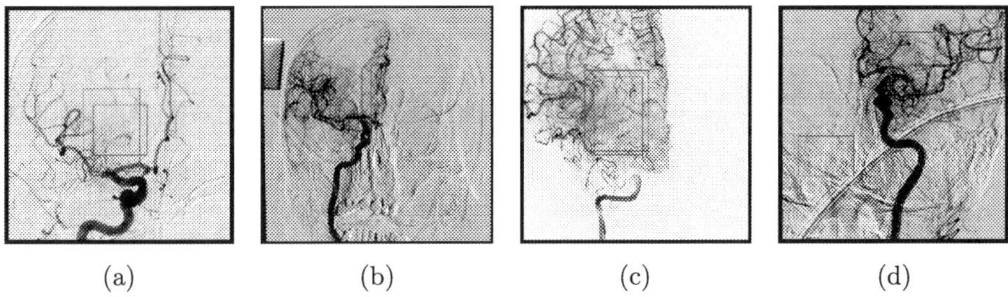

Fig. 4. Example outputs (green) and ground truths (red) for enhanced input images (Color figure online)

3.3 Output Examples and Error Analysis

To further aid the interpretation of the results, some example outputs are shown in Fig. 4. Note that in this figure, the input images were enhanced, but the bounding boxes are shown over the not-enhanced images. In Figs. 4a, b, c, there is a slight discrepancy between the size of the predicted and ground-truth bounding boxes. The clearer parts of the blush seem more easily recognized, which is observable in Fig. 4c. Therefore, it is likely that blush is often correctly classified as such but only the clearer parts. This results in no full overlap which explains some of the imperfections in the metrics listed in Table 1.

It should also be noted that these metrics are the average over the test set. The test set contains clinical data with its imperfections. As can be seen in Fig. 4d, noise and motion artifacts may degrade image quality, which is harder for the model. It might be due to the similarity between the textural features of the blush and noise/motion artifacts. This limitation on the performance shows that the proposed system at this stage is not yet robust to all imperfections present in clinical data, e.g. noise and motion artifacts.

The cases in which no overlap is found are scored by 0 in both similarity metrics. As the means are considered over the test set, these cases weigh down the average considerably. Therefore, if more robustness to these imperfections can be introduced, the metric scores should increase.

4 Conclusions

Perfusion in the lenticulostriate territory deserves attention after ischemic stroke as no collateral blood flow reaches this region. In this paper, the first-ever segmentation of the blush in the lenticulostriate territory is proposed. The segmentations of the blush and the hemisphere are explored using deep-learning methods. The ratio between these segmentations is a sample quantification of the blush.

Ideas for future research include retraining the network on larger datasets, as the model performs less well in the presence of imperfections in clinical data. Larger datasets containing more noise and motion artifacts should aid robustness. Furthermore, only the anteroposterior view is considered in this paper. As X-ray imaging shows the result of a projection through a volume, information in the depth dimension is lost and information in a 2D image is susceptible to the angle under which it was taken. Therefore, a more complete view of the lenticulostriate territory may be obtained by also including a sagittal view. As blush is considered in this paper, further research into how well blush correlates with perfusion and cerebral blood flow is required. Furthermore, only the information in the DSA images is used without considering the timing of the images. The effect of transit time delay on the method should be systematically investigated in future research. Also, a closer inspection of the blush is of interest. The branches from which the perforating arteries arise should be incorporated into the method, which may allow compartmentation of the blush.

The overall results presented in this paper are promising, but difficulties like noise and motion artifacts seem to be hurdles in the way of clinical application. If more research resolves these hurdles, the segmentation of the blush in the lenticulostriate territory forms the basis from which quantitative analysis can progress. This can ultimately be used to evaluate treatment effectivity, contribute toward prognosis prediction, and tailor further care for stroke patients.

References

1. Asif, M., et al.: Intracranial hemorrhage detection using parallel deep convolutional models and boosting mechanism. Diagnostics **13**(4), 652 (2023)
2. Decavel, P., Vuillier, F., Moulin, T.: Lenticulostriate infarction. Manif. Stroke **30**, 115–119 (2012)
3. Ertuğrul, Ö.F., Akıl, M.F.: Detecting hemorrhage types and bounding box of hemorrhage by deep learning. Biomed. Signal Process. Control **71**, 103085 (2022)
4. Girshick, R.: Fast R-CNN (2015)
5. He, K., Zhang, X., Ren, S., Sun, J.: Deep residual learning for image recognition. In: Proceedings of the IEEE Conference on Computer Vision and Pattern Recognition, pp. 770–778 (2016)
6. Hendriks, E.J., Klostranec, J.M., Krings, T.: Digital subtraction angiography. In: Mannil, M., Winklhofer, S.F.-X. (eds.) Neuroimaging Techniques in Clinical Practice, pp. 23–30. Springer, Cham (2020). https://doi.org/10.1007/978-3-030-48419-4_3

7. Herpich, F., Rincon, F.: Management of acute ischemic stroke. Crit. Care Med. **48**(11), 1654 (2020)
8. Liu, W., et al.: SSD: single shot multibox detector. In: Leibe, B., Matas, J., Sebe, N., Welling, M. (eds.) ECCV 2016. LNCS, vol. 9905, pp. 21–37. Springer, Cham (2016). https://doi.org/10.1007/978-3-319-46448-0_2
9. Paul, S., Candelario-Jalil, E.: Emerging neuroprotective strategies for the treatment of ischemic stroke: an overview of clinical and preclinical studies. Exp. Neurol. **335**, 113518 (2021)
10. Rahmany, I., Guetari, R., Khlifa, N.: A fully automatic based deep learning approach for aneurysm detection in DSA images. In: 2018 IEEE International Conference on Image Processing, Applications and Systems (IPAS), pp. 303–307. IEEE (2018)
11. Rzepliński, R., et al.: Standard clinical computed tomography fails to precisely visualise presence, course and branching points of deep cerebral perforators. Folia Morphol. **82**(1), 37–41 (2021)
12. Su, R., et al.: Spatio-temporal deep learning for automatic detection of intracranial vessel perforation in digital subtraction angiography during endovascular thrombectomy. Med. Image Anal. **77**, 102377 (2022)
13. The MathWorks Inc.: Matlab: imadjust (2023). https://nl.mathworks.com/help/images/ref/imadjust.html
14. The MathWorks Inc.: Matlab: object detection using SSD deep learning (2023). https://nl.mathworks.com/help/vision/ug/object-detection-using-single-shot-detector.html
15. Weber, M., Perona, P.: Caltech cars 1999 (2022). https://doi.org/10.22002/D1.20084
16. Wei, N., Zhang, X., An, J., Zhuo, Y., Zhang, Z.: A processing pipeline for quantifying lenticulostriate artery vascular volume in subcortical nuclei. Front. Neurol. **12**, 700476 (2021)
17. Xu, X., et al.: Characterization of lenticulostriate arteries and its associations with vascular risk factors in community-dwelling elderly. Front. Aging Neurosci. **13**, 685571 (2021)

Multimodal Deep Learning for Functional Outcome Prediction in Endovascular Therapy

Frank te Nijenhuis[1(✉)], Ruisheng Su[1], Pieter Jan van Doormaal[1], Jeannette Hofmeijer[2,3], Jasper Martens[4], Wim van Zwam[5], Aad van der Lugt[1], and Theo van Walsum[1]

[1] Department of Radiology and Nuclear Medicine, Erasmus MC, University Medical Center Rotterdam, Rotterdam, The Netherlands
f.tenijenhuis@erasmusmc.nl

[2] Clinical Neurophysiology, MIRA Institute for Biomedical Technology and Technical Medicine, University of Twente, Enschede, The Netherlands

[3] Department of Neurology, Rijnstate Hospital, Arnhem, The Netherlands

[4] Department of Radiology and Nuclear Medicine, Rijnstate Hospital, Arnhem, The Netherlands

[5] Department of Radiology and Nuclear Medicine, Maastricht UMC, Cardiovascular Research Institute Maastricht, Maastricht, The Netherlands

Abstract. The efficacy of endovascular therapy (EVT) in large vessel occlusion (LVO) of the anterior circulation depends on adequate patient selection. Patients can be selected based on their predicted functional outcome after EVT. Using a dataset composed of 1929 patients, we compare the functional outcome prediction performance of clinical baseline models, including the clinically validated MR PREDICTS decision tool, with an imaging based pipeline and a multimodal approach. The predicted outcome measure is dichotomized modified Rankin Scale score 90 days after mechanical thrombectomy. Binary classifier performance is quantified using Area-Under the receiver operating characteristic Curve (AUC). Combining clinical features with information extracted from CTA images does not significantly improve the performance of functional outcome prediction methods compared to the baseline model. This multimodal approach can however replace radiologically derived biomarkers, as its performance is non-inferior.

Keywords: Stroke · Deep Learning · Artificial Intelligence · Functional Outcome Prediction · Mechanical Thrombectomy · Endovascular Therapy · Med3D · MR CLEAN Registry · MR PREDICTS

Supplementary Information The online version contains supplementary material available at https://doi.org/10.1007/978-3-031-76160-7_14.

U. Baid et al. (Eds.): BrainLes 2023/SWITCH 2023, LNCS 14668, pp. 144–153, 2024.
https://doi.org/10.1007/978-3-031-76160-7_14

1 Introduction

In recent years, mechanical thrombectomy, also referred to as endovascular therapy (EVT), has emerged as an effective procedure for the treatment of acute ischemic stroke (AIS) in patients with a large vessel occlusion (LVO) [3–5,8,13]. Although recent developments indicate that EVT is feasible and worthwhile in most patients, even in a delayed treatment setting [14,21], adequate functional outcome prediction systems may prove useful by providing the patient with personalized prognostic information based on their parameters. Furthermore, investigating functional outcome prediction may provide insight into the interaction between the underlying disease process and the therapeutic outcome after EVT.

Multiple scoring methods have been developed to prognosticate functional outcome after EVT, using 90-day modified Rankin Scale (mRS90) as the outcome variable. As these methods are based on traditional statistical techniques they are not equipped to extract information directly from radiological images. Additionally, they often require radiological image biomarker information, which necessitates an arduous process of expert annotation, complicated by the oftentimes high degree of inter-observer variability [11].

AI based decision support systems might be of added benefit in this regard, by automating the functional outcome prediction process.

We hypothesize that information encoded in baseline imaging, as performed for stroke patients prior to EVT, can be extracted using deep learning based methods. A deep learning model that has been trained to effectively predict functional outcome after EVT can be utilized to inform clinical decision making.

1.1 Related Work

Recent research has focused on predicting functional outcome using a combination of clinical features as well as imaging features extracted using deep learning based methods. Table 1 summarizes previous results in this area. Zihni et al. used a combined pipeline with a Convolutional Neural Network (CNN) to extract imaging features as well as an MLP to process clinical data. The imaging data consisted of 3D volumes of TOF-MRA images. They show that an end-to-end multimodal pipeline integrating neuroimaging and clinical data leads to the best performance when predicting dichotomized mRS90 [22]. Bacchi et al. predict dichotomized mRS90 using several CNN and MLP based models, focusing on a combination of clinical and imaging data. For the imaging data, Non-Contrast CT (NCCT) scans are used. The best performing model is a combination of CNN and MLP [2]. Samak et al. also use NCCT imaging data, in combination with clinical information [17]. Hilbert et al. [11] and De Graaf [10] both successfully use deep learning models trained on CT Angiography (CTA) images, showing that these images also contain relevant information with regards to functional outcome prediction.

1.2 Contributions

We investigate a multimodal framework, combining processing of clinical features with the output of an image analysis backbone. We compare the performance of a

Table 1. Earlier work in mRS prediction after 90 days. TOF-MRA: Time Of Flight Magnetic Resonance Angiography, NCCT: Non-Contrast CT, CTA: CT Angiography. [a]Subgroup contains mRS90 score of 0–1.

Paper	Image Modality	AUC Multimodal	Total Dataset Size	Size of mRS90 0-2 Subgroup (%)
Zihni et al. [22]	TOF-MRA	0.76	313	87 (27.8 %)
Bacchi et al. [2]	NCCT	0.75	204	113 (55.4%)[a]
Samak et al. [17]	NCCT	0.75	500	127 (25.4%)
Hilbert et al. [11]	CTA	0.71	1526	463 (35.6%)
De Graaf [10]	CTA	0.78	1000	417 (41.7%)

state-of-the-art medical image processing model with clinical baseline models, to investigate whether functional outcome prediction performance can be improved. Training is performed on a dataset containing CTA images as well as clinical features of 1929 patients, which, to the best of our knowledge, is the largest dataset on which such an effort has been undertaken so far.

2 Methods

We investigated three modeling frameworks in predicting dichotomized mRS90. A schematic overview of these processing pipelines is provided in Fig. 1.

The simplest framework is the *clinical model*, which takes input features as used by the MR PREDICTS model [20], displayed in Table 2, and passes these through a Multilayer Perceptron (MLP) set up as a classifier, or a Linear Regression (LR) model. We divide the input features into clinical and radiological features, where clinical features are derived from patient data, and radiological features are acquired by a radiologist manually inspecting images. Input features are shown in Table 2.

The *imaging model* consists of the Med3D deep learning model, which we modify (see Sect. 2.1) to take CTA scans as input [7]. A final linear layer maps the 64 output features of the modified Med3D to a single unnormalized output value.

The third framework we consider is the *combined model*, which concatenates the outputs of the *clinical* model with the output of the *imaging* model and passes the combined output to a fully connected layer. The final output is a single classification node.

2.1 Med3D Modifications

Med3D is a residual CNN specifically designed for medical image analysis. It was originally intended for segmentation purposes, but it can be reconfigured as a classification network. It consists of a modified ResNet backbone with an upsampling branch. The ResNet backbone was modified by changing the number

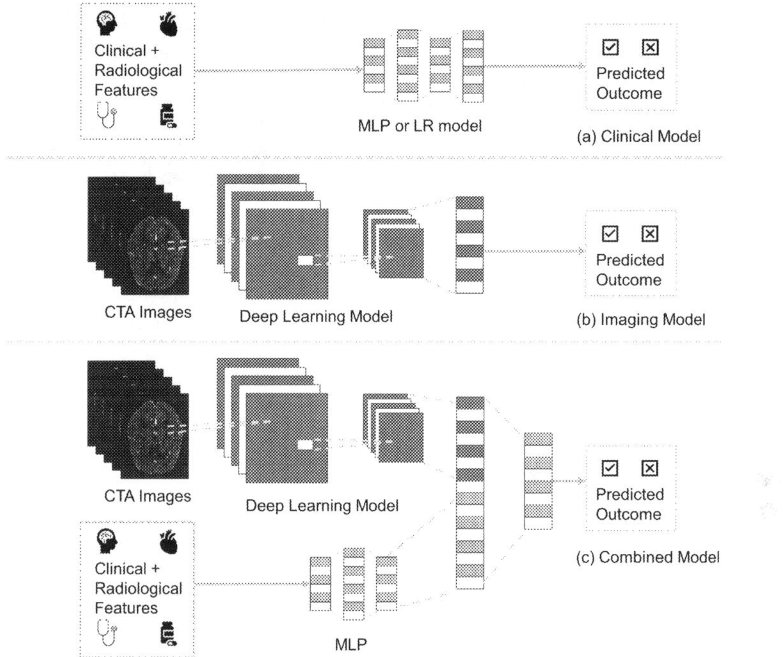

Fig. 1. Schematic overview of the unimodal and multimodal architectures. (a) shows the unimodal clinical model, which processes clinical (and radiological) features, but not information extracted directly from CTA images, using either an MLP (as depicted) or a LR model. (b) is a schematic representation of the unimodal imaging model, which uses Med3D to directly infer functional outcome from the CTA images. Finally, (c) is a multimodal approach, combining the previous architectures by concatenating the outputs. DLM: Deep Learning Model. MLP: Multi-Layer Perceptron. FCL: Fully-Connected Layer. LR: Linear Regression.

of input channels from three to one, by expanding the 2D convolution operations to 3D convolutions, by setting the stride in layers three and four of the network to one to remove downsampling, and by using dilated convolutions in the downstream convolutional layers. We opt for the ResNet50 as a backbone for Med3D. We initialize the Med3D architecture using the weights which were stored after training on the 3D segmentation dataset as described in [7]. We further modify the Med3D network by replacing the final segmentation layer with an average pooling layer followed by a linear layer mapping to 64 features.

3 Data

We use the MR CLEAN registry, which is an ongoing prospective observational study involving 17 centers in the Netherlands. For each patient the dataset contains demographic information, information about clinical parameters and patient outcomes. The patient features we use as predictors are derived from the

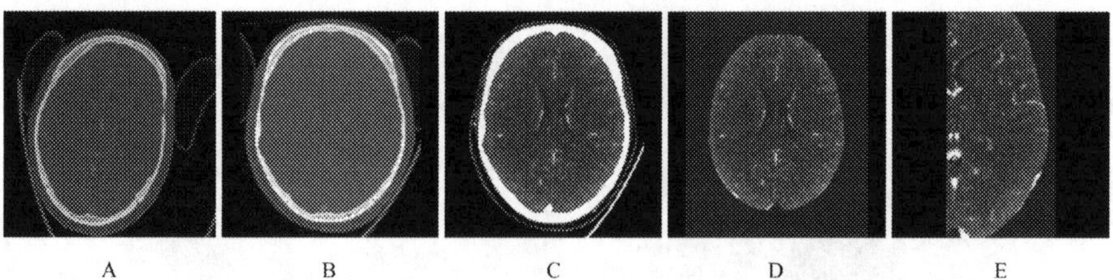

Fig. 2. Illustration of the preprocessing pipeline, from left to right. A: original image, B: after registration to brain atlas, C: after normalization and clipping, D: after brain masking, E: after midline mirroring (to align all occlusions to the left hemisphere) and hemisphere masking.

MR PREDICTS clinical decision tool and are displayed in Table 2. The accompanying preoperative CTA scan is also available for each included patient, as well as the mRS90 score.

In total, we selected 1929 patients from MR CLEAN registries 1, 2 & 3. For detailed information regarding the preprocessing steps, we refer to the supplementary material. An illustration of the preprocessing pipeline is provided in Fig. 2. The selected scans were registered to a brain atlas using the ANTs software [1]. The construction of this atlas is described in [16].

In both subsets, the quality of the scans was assessed using visual inspection, after image registration. Images were rejected if registration failed, if the brain coverage was insufficient, if there were visible artefacts or if the wrong procedure was performed. In total, 1929 patients were included. The clinical features are summarized in Table 2.

Clinical data are normalized between zero and one to facilitate handling by the neural networks. Missing data were imputed for all independent variables using Multiple Imputation by Chained Equations (MICE, [18]) with a Gaussian Mixture estimator.

4 Experiments and Results

An independent test set is obtained by randomly sampling 10% of the data ($n = 192$), the remaining data is divided using a stratified five-fold cross validation procedure.

Average validation performance is displayed in Table 3. ROC curves are produced by applying the best validated version of each classifier on the held-out test set. Table 4 shows the test set performance for the models with the best performance on the validation sets. DeLong's test for comparison of ROC curves reveals that there is no statistically significant difference between LR trained on the radiological features (AUC = 0.57, $n = 192$) and the Med3D model trained on CTA images only (AUC = 0.65, $z = 1.19$, $p = 0.235$). Similarly, no statistically

Table 2. Baseline characteristics for the patient, using the unimputed, unnormalized original data. Glucose in mmol/l, BP: Blood Pressure in mmHg. ICA: internal carotid artery. M1-3: branches of the middle cerebral artery. [a]radiologically derived features.

Feature	MR CLEAN Registry 1, 2 & 3 (n = 1929)	MR CLEAN Registry mRS90 0-2 (n = 813, 42.1%)	MR CLEAN Registry mRS90 3-6 (n = 1116, 57.9%)
Median Age (IQR)	72 (63-80)	69 (57-76)	76 (67-83)
Male % (n)	52% (1008)	57% (465)	49% (543)
Median ASPECTS (IQR)[a]	9 (8-10)	9 (8-10)	9 (8-10)
DM % (n)	17% (329)	11% (88)	22 % (241)
Mean Glucose (std)	7.40 (2.48)	7.01 (2.11)	7.70 (2.68)
Median baseline NIHSS (IQR)	16 (11-19)	13 (8-17)	17(13-21)
Median pre-stroke mRS (IQR)	0 (0-1)	0 (0-0)	0 (0-2)
Intravenous Alteplase % (n)	64% (1230)	71% (571)	59% (659)
Occlusion location % (n)[a]			
ICA	24.00 % (463)	19.80 % (161)	27.06% (302)
M1	57.02% (1100)	59.04 % (480)	55.56% (620)
M2	18.40 % (355)	20.66 % (168)	16.76% (187)
M3	0.10% (2)	0.25% (2)	0.00% (0)
Collateral score % (n)[a]			
Absent	4.56% (88)	1.85 % (15)	6.54 % (73)
<50%	36.13% (697)	28.17 % (229)	41.94 % (468)
>50<100%	38.00% (733)	41.94 % (341)	35.13% (392)
100%	20.11% (388)	26.69 % (217)	15.32% (171)
Median Systolic BP (IQR)	150 (132-167)	147 (130-163)	150 (135-170)
Median time-to-groin (IQR)	185 (136-265)	173 (130-250)	195 (145-275)

significant difference was found between LR and the MLP (AUC = 0.57, $z = 0.36$, $p = 0.714$).

Comparing LR trained on the clinical features only (AUC = 0.75, n = 192) reveals no statistically significant difference with the multimodal model trained on CTA images and clinical features (AUC = 0.73, $z = 0.72$, $p = 0.471$). Similar comparison between LR and the MLP (AUC = 0.74, $z = 0.89$, $p = 0.373$) again yields no statistically significant difference.

Finally, comparing the performance of the MR PREDICTS clinical decision tool [20] on the combined radiological and clinical features (AUC = 0.77, n = 192) with the multimodal model does not lead to a statistically significant difference (AUC = 0.73, $z = 1.12$, $p = 0.263$). The MR PREDICTS model performs comparably to the MLP (AUC = 0.76, $z = 0.35$, $p = 0.721$). ROC curves for this final comparison are displayed in Fig. 3.

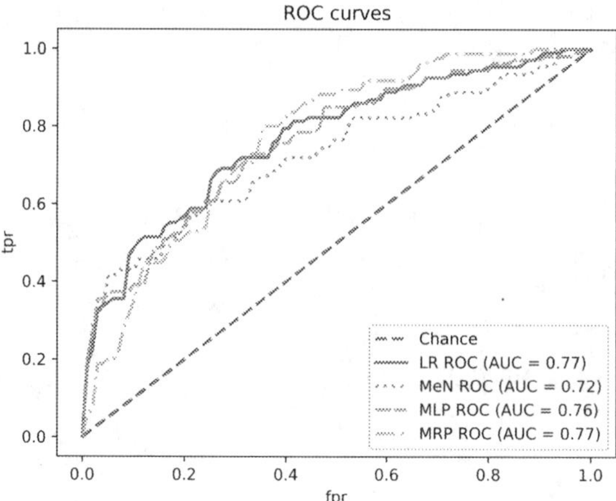

Fig. 3. Receiver-Operating Characteristic (ROC) curves showing performance on the test set for the Image + Clinical + Radiological case. LR: Logistic Regression, MeN: Med3D, MRP: MR PREDICTS, tpr: true positive rate, fpr: false positive rate.

5 Discussion

We have investigated whether multimodal deep learning can be used to predict functional outcome after mechanical thrombectomy in patients suffering from LVO of the anterior circulation, and demonstrated that it achieves comparable performance to the MR PREDICTS clinical decision making tool. Inclusion of pre-processed imaging data using an end-to-end deep learning model does not, however, significantly improve performance compared to conventional statistical methods.

When comparing the performance of the imaging framework with logistic regression trained on the radiological features, we see a moderate (but not statistically significant) increase in performance. These results imply that end-to-end deep learning models can extract latent information from imaging which is at least partially complementary to the information contained in clinical and radiological features. While deep learning does not improve functional outcome prediction performance, the results do suggest a potential role in replacing the radiologically derived parameters.

These results are comparable to results obtained in related work, where similar deep learning methods are applied on different imaging modalities to predict mRS90, see also Sect. 1.1, as well as Table 1. The fact that multiple authors employing different deep learning methods on distinct imaging modalities, have not been able to demonstrate significant improvement over conventional methods suggests that functional outcome prediction is a challenging problem.

In this study we investigated the practicality of neural networks when analyzing CTA images. One potential new avenue of research would be to investigate whether addition of non-contrast CT, CT-perfusion or MRI (DWI) information,

Table 3. Average 5-fold validation performance of each classifier. Med3D shows the best average performance for each data category. [a]: These models cannot handle image inputs, so they only use clinical and radiological variables. In the case of the "Image only" dataset, they only received radiological features. See also Table 2 for the radiologically derived features.

		Image only	Image + Clinical	Image + Clinical + Radiological
LR[a]	AUC (± s.d)	0,58 (± 0,002)	0,75 (± 0,002)	0,70 (± 0,009)
	Accuracy (± s.d)	0,53 (± 0,005)	0,53 (± 0,005)	0,71 (± 0,009)
MLP[a]	AUC (± s.d)	0,62 (± 0,031)	0,79 (± 0,028)	0,74 (± 0,047)
	Accuracy (± s.d)	0,61 (± 0,016)	0,73 (± 0,015)	0,72 (± 0,056)
Med3D	AUC (± s.d)	**0,68 (± 0,036)**	**0,82 (± 0,131)**	**0,88 (± 0,039)**
	Accuracy (± s.d)	**0,88 (± 0,082)**	**0,85 (± 0,120)**	**0,92 (± 0,030)**

Table 4. Test set performance of the models with the best validation performance. [a]: see Table 3.

		Image only	Image + Clinical	Image + Clinical + Radiological
LR[a]	AUC	0.57	**0.75**	**0.77**
MLP[a]	AUC	0.57	0.74	0.76
Med3D	AUC	**0.65**	0.73	0.73

for instance as a different input channel to the classifier, would yield better results.

It is not yet clear to what extent features extracted from the images are complementary to the clinical and radiological features, future work should investigate which features are most relevant to the classifiers, and why. One potential way to do this is by regressing on the MR PREDICTS variables using the raw features extracted by the imaging classifiers.

A potential limitation of this work is the fact that we have only studied patients who underwent EVT, which makes it difficult to draw conclusions about the performance of these methods when presented with patients not undergoing this treatment. This also means that these methods are not directly clinically applicable, instead they should serve as a basis for future research.

6 Conclusion

We set out to investigate the potential usefulness of deep learning methods in improving functional outcome prediction after mechanical thrombectomy in stroke patients. Results did not indicate a significant performance improvement of multimodal, end-to-end deep learning methods, which combine imaging data with patient features, compared to conventional statistical methods based only on patient features. Future research must reveal whether multimodal deep learning techniques can be of concrete clinical value.

Acknowledgements. We want to thank the MR CLEAN Registry investigators for their contributions.

Sources of Funding. The MR CLEAN Registry was funded and carried out by the Erasmus University Medical Centre, Amsterdam University Medical Centers, location AMC, and Maastricht University Medical Centre. The study was additionally funded by the Applied Scientific Institute for Neuromodulation (Toegepast Wetenschappelijk Instituut voor Neuromodulatie [TWIN]).

References

1. Avants, B., Tustison, N., Song, G.: Advanced normalization tools (ANTS). Insight J., 1–35 (2008). https://doi.org/10.54294/uvnhin
2. Bacchi, S., Zerner, T., Oakden-Rayner, L., Kleinig, T., Patel, S., Jannes, J.: Deep learning in the prediction of ischaemic stroke thrombolysis functional outcomes: a pilot study. Acad. Radiol. **27**(2), e19–e23 (2020). https://doi.org/10.1016/j.acra.2019.03.015. https://www.sciencedirect.com/science/article/pii/S1076633219301746
3. Beumer, D., Staals, J., Hofmeijer, J., Boiten, J., et al.: A randomized trial of intraarterial treatment for acute ischemic stroke. N. Engl. J. Med. (2015). https://doi.org/10.1056/nejmoa1411587
4. Broderick, J.P., Palesch, Y.Y., Demchuk, A.M., Yeatts, S.D., et al.: Endovascular therapy after intravenous t-PA versus t-PA alone for stroke. N. Engl. J. Med. (2013). https://doi.org/10.1056/nejmoa1214300
5. Campbell, B.C., Churilov, L., Yassi, N., Yan, B., et al.: Endovascular therapy for ischemic stroke with perfusion-imaging selection. N. Engl. J. Med. (2015). https://doi.org/10.1056/nejmoa1414792
6. Chen, A., Chow, A., Davidson, A., DCunha, A., et al.: Developments in MLflow: a system to accelerate the machine learning lifecycle. In: Proceedings of the Fourth International Workshop on Data Management for End-to-End Machine Learning, DEEM 2020. Association for Computing Machinery, New York (2020). https://doi.org/10.1145/3399579.3399867
7. Chen, S., Ma, K., Zheng, Y.: Med3D: transfer learning for 3D medical image analysis. CoRR abs/1904.00625 (2019). http://arxiv.org/abs/1904.00625
8. Ciccone, A., Valvassori, L., Nichelatti, M., Sgoifo, A., et al.: Endovascular treatment for acute ischemic stroke. N. Engl. J. Med. (2013). https://doi.org/10.1056/nejmoa1213701
9. Falcon, W., et al.: Pytorch lightning. GitHub. https://github.com/PyTorchLightning/pytorch-lightning (2019)
10. de Graaf, S.: Automated functional outcome prediction in stroke using combined imaging and clinical parameters. Master's thesis, TU Delft, the Netherlands (2022). https://repository.tudelft.nl/islandora/object/uuid%3Ab6b126e7-b589-428a-a86a-f3d04cf9f85c?collection=education

11. Hilbert, A., Ramos, L., van Os, H., Olabarriaga, S., et al.: Data-efficient deep learning of radiological image data for outcome prediction after endovascular treatment of patients with acute ischemic stroke. Comput. Biol. Med. **115**, 103516 (2019). https://doi.org/10.1016/j.compbiomed.2019.103516. https://www.sciencedirect.com/science/article/pii/S0010482519303786
12. Loshchilov, I., Hutter, F.: Fixing weight decay regularization in Adam. CoRR abs/1711.05101 (2017). http://arxiv.org/abs/1711.05101
13. McCarthy, D.J., Diaz, A., Sheinberg, D., Snelling, B.M., et al.: Long-term outcomes of mechanical thrombectomy for stroke: a meta-analysis. Sci. World J. (2019). https://doi.org/10.1155/2019/7403104
14. Olthuis, S.G.H., Pirson, F.A.V., Pinckaers, F.M.E., Hinsenveld, W.H., et al.: Endovascular treatment versus no endovascular treatment after 6–24 h in patients with ischaemic stroke and collateral flow on CT angiography (MR CLEAN-LATE) in the Netherlands: a multicentre, open-label, blinded-endpoint, randomised, controlled, phase 3 trial. Lancet **401**(10385), 1371–1380 (2023)
15. Paszke, A., Gross, S., Massa, F., Lerer, A., et al.: PyTorch: an imperative style, high-performance deep learning library. CoRR abs/1912.01703 (2019). http://arxiv.org/abs/1912.01703
16. Peter, R., Emmer, B.J., van Es, A.C., van Walsum, T.: Cortical and vascular probability maps for analysis of human brain in computed tomography images. In: 2017 IEEE 14th International Symposium on Biomedical Imaging (ISBI 2017), pp. 1141–1145 (2017). https://doi.org/10.1109/ISBI.2017.7950718
17. Samak, Z.A., Clatworthy, P., Mirmehdi, M.: Prediction of thrombectomy functional outcomes using multimodal data. In: Papież, B.W., Namburete, A.I.L., Yaqub, M., Noble, J.A. (eds.) MIUA 2020. CCIS, vol. 1248, pp. 267–279. Springer, Cham (2020). https://doi.org/10.1007/978-3-030-52791-4_21
18. Van Buuren, S., Oudshoorn, K.: Flexible multivariate imputation by MICE. TNO, Leiden (1999)
19. Van Rossum, G., Drake, F.L.: Python 3 Reference Manual. CreateSpace, Scotts Valley (2009)
20. Venema, E., Roozenbeek, B., Mulder, M.J., Brown, S., et al.: Prediction of outcome and endovascular treatment benefit: validation and update of the MR PREDICTS decision tool. Stroke **52**(9), 2764–2772 (2021). https://doi.org/10.1161/STROKEAHA.120.032935
21. Wardlaw, J.M.: Even more benefit with endovascular treatment for patients with acute ischaemic stroke: MR CLEAN-LATE. Lancet **401**(10385), 1317–1319 (2023)
22. Zihni., E., Madai., V., Khalil., A., Galinovic., I., et al.: Multimodal fusion strategies for outcome prediction in stroke. In: Proceedings of the 13th International Joint Conference on Biomedical Engineering Systems and Technologies - HEALTHINF, pp. 421–428. INSTICC, SciTePress (2020). https://doi.org/10.5220/0008957304210428

Framework to Generate Perfusion Map from CT and CTA Images in Patients with Acute Ischemic Stroke: A Longitudinal and Cross-Sectional Study

Chayanin Tangwiriysakul[1(✉)], Pedro Borges[1], Stefano Moriconi[1,3], Paul Wright[1], Yee-Haur Mah[4], James Teo[4], Parashkev Nachev[2], Sebastien Ourselin[1], and M. Jorge Cardoso[1]

[1] School of Biomedical Engineering and Imaging Sciences, King's College London, London SE1 7EU, UK
chayanin.tangwiriyasakul@kcl.ac.uk

[2] UCL Queen Square Institute of Neurology, University College London, London WC1B 5EH, UK

[3] Support Center for Advanced Neuroimaging (SCAN), University Institute of Diagnostic and Interventional Radiology, University of Bern, Inselspital, Bern University Hospital, 3010 Bern, Switzerland

[4] King's College Hospital NHS Foundation Trust, Denmark Hill, London SE5 9RS, UK

Abstract. Stroke is a leading cause of disability and death. Effective treatment decisions require early and informative vascular imaging. 4D perfusion imaging is ideal but rarely available within the first hour after stroke, whereas plain CT and CTA usually are. Hence, we propose a framework to extract a predicted perfusion map (PPM) derived from CT and CTA images. In all eighteen patients, we found significantly high spatial similarity (with average Spearman's correlation = 0.7893) between our predicted perfusion map (PPM) and the T-max map derived from 4D-CTP. Voxelwise correlations between the PPM and National Institutes of Health Stroke Scale (NIHSS) subscores for L/R hand motor, gaze, and language on a large cohort of 2,110 subjects reliably mapped symptoms to expected infarct locations. Therefore our PPM could serve as an alternative for 4D perfusion imaging, if the latter is unavailable, to investigate blood perfusion in the first hours after hospital admission.

1 Introduction

Stroke is one of the leading causes of disability or death. About 15 million people suffer from stroke worldwide per year [1]. The first hour after admission to a stroke unit is considered the golden hour, in which the patients who receive suitable treatments have a higher chance of avoiding long-term brain damage [2]. The benefit of receiving proper treatment within this golden hour in stroke was seen in all age groups [3]. Thus, all efforts should be made to give all patients the

U. Baid et al. (Eds.): BrainLes 2023/SWITCH 2023, LNCS 14668, pp. 154–162, 2024.
https://doi.org/10.1007/978-3-031-76160-7_15

most suitable treatment within that time frame. Currently, 4-dimensional CT or MR perfusion imaging (4D-CTP) is used to investigate blood flow through the brain vessels and ultimately predict infarct location [4]. However, its acquisition process is complex. On top of that, 4D-CTP requires specialised software to compute clinically useful 3D maps of cerebral blood flow, cerebral blood volume, or time-to-maximum (T-max). Taken together, they limit the number of patients eligible for 4D-CTP. In contrast, plain CT and CT angiography (CTA) are routinely acquired on admission to the stroke pathway and so are available earlier and for more patients.

As a neurovascular disease, the loss of brain function after blood vessel blockages cause stroke onset. Three cerebral regions can be defined after stroke onset: the ischemic core, the penumbra and the oligemic region. The ischemic core is the brain area with cerebral blood flow between 4.8 to 8.4 mL/100 g per minute [5,6]. Unlike the penumbra and the oligemic region, depletion of blood flow in the ischemic core lead to cell death and cause permanent brain damage. Understanding cerebral blood flow using a perfusion map is one of the keys to helping provide patients with proper treatments or predict possible brain damage.

This study presents a framework to generate a predicted perfusion map (PPM) derived from CT and CTA in the first hours after admission as an alternative to 4D-CTP. We validated our PPM using both longitudinal and cross-sectional analyses. The former was done by comparing the spatial similarity between our PPM and the T-max map derived from 4D-CTP in eighteen subjects. The latter was done by testing the relationship between the PPM and National Institutes of Health Stroke Scale (NIHSS) subscores, which is a standardised series of bedside tests used to assess the severity of stroke symptoms, in a large cohort of 2,110 patients. In summary, we have developed a deployable framework and validated it with clinical data to show it produces images containing similar information about cerebral perfusion to 4D-CTP.

2 Method

2.1 Data Set

We selected a continuous cohort of patients admitted to the stroke unit at King's College Hospital on the basis of having both CT and CTA and evaluation with the NIHSS. Note that right after being admitted to the A&E unit, NIHSS are evaluated in every patient. Later within 5 to 20 min, a CT and CTA are acquired. Inclusion criteria were met by 2,110 patients (mean [SD] age = 68.8 [15.9] years, female = 936 [44%]). Of these, eighteen had 4D-CTP (mean [SD] age = 61.9 [13.3] years, female = 8 [44%]).

2.2 Data Pre-processing and Estimation of Predicted Perfusion Map

Each patient's images were prepared using SPM12 [7]. We coregistered the CT to the CTA, computed affine registration of the CT to MNI space, and applied this to both, reslicing images to $1 \times 1 \times 1$ mm resolution. The prepared images were inputs in VTrails [8,9]. In this study, we only run the first two steps of VTrails: (1) digital subtraction image pre-processing and (2) vascular contrast enhancement and seeds detection. In step 1, we created a digitally subtracted image (DSA) by composite registration (Affine + BSpline) with CTA as a reference image and CT as the moving image, followed by subtraction of CT from CTA. Later the DSA image was normalised by its maximum value. In step 2, we extracted seed points from the vascular contrast-enhanced version of the DSA [8,9]. In this step, we first applied a gradient anisotropic filter to the DSA image as in Perona-Malik [10,11]. The aim of this filter is to suppress noise while preserving edges (of the vascular structure in our case). We call this filtered DSA image or VSP. We then binarised the VSP image to segment the vessels. Any voxel in the VSP image with an intensity higher than 0.2 is considered a part of the vessel. Note that 0.2 is the default parameter in VTrails [8,12]. The binarised VSP was later converted into the skeleton image (SKEL) using itkBinaryThinningImagheFilter3D in ITK [13]. The skeleton depicts the centreline of the vascular structure. itkBinaryThinningImagheFilter3D was developed based on Lee et al. [14], which is a 3D decision tree-based algorithm aiming to thin the binary image. Any voxel along the skeleton image with its corresponding value in the VSP image at the same (x, y, z) location greater than its 75th percentile (VTrails' default parameter) was considered a seed point.

The DSA and Seed images were later used to estimate time-of-arrival at each voxel. A fast marching algorithm was used to estimate the time-of-arrival at each voxel with the seed points as the source and the DSA as the speed potential matrix [15]. The fast-marching algorithm is a special case of Dijkstra's algorithm [16]. The aim of a fast-marching algorithm is to extract a minimal geodesic path by minimising an energy function weighted by an image speed potential connecting any possible path between two points [8,16]. In our study, all the seed points are located along the centerline of the lumen contour. The velocity profile is highest along the centreline and monotonically decreases away from the centre [17]. Thus our seed points located along the centreline are chosen to act as the source to supply blood/oxygen to its closest neighbouring brain areas (in our study, we assume the continuation of blood flow within the vessels). Each seed point will propagate through the anisotropic medium (in our case, the speed potential matrix). The voxelwise image of time-of-arrival comprises the PPM. Since the DSA was normalised between 0 to 1 (where the voxel intensity inside the vascular structure was higher than its surrounding tissue), the PPM is unitless. A higher voxel value reflects a longer time taken for blood to perfuse the location, hence a higher risk of ischemia at that voxel. Figure 1 depicts all steps to estimate the PPM from CT and CTA. We run our scripts using MATLAB2020a on an Intel(R) Core(TM) i9-9900K computer. For each subject, it took 539 s (SD = 49 s) to proprocess CT/CTA images, run VTrails and estimate PPM.

2.3 Longitudinal Analysis

In eighteen subjects, a 4D-CTP image was acquired. The RAPID-AI software (https://www.rapidai.com/, California USA) was used to derive a Time-to-maximum (T-max) image from the 4D-CTP image. T-max is a parameter of the modelled perfusion representing the time for contrast to reach each voxel from the proximal large artery. It is commonly used to predict infarction maps [18, 19]. In our study, each exported T-max volume was first converted into a greyscale volume and later coregistered to the PPM using SPM-12. To enhance the visibility of the infarct core, we applied a Gaussian filter with a kernel size of 10 voxels to both the exported T-max and the PPM as suggested by Campbell et al. [20]. Finally, we estimated a Spearman's rank correlation coefficient between the exported T-max map with the PPM to assess the level of similarity. In this study, we used Spearman's rank correlation coefficient because the unit of the Rapid T-max map and our PPM did not match but are correlated. Furthermore, we evaluated if the spatial similarity between our PPM and T-max correlated with age. In this study, we chose the T-max map as a benchmark since it is used to predict the final infarct size and functional outcomes in patients with ischemic stroke [21].

2.4 Cross-Sectional Analysis

The NIHSS is a standardised series of bedside tests used to assess the severity of stroke symptoms. It comprises eleven sub-scores such as level of consciousness and limb mobility [22]. In this study, we focused on the four primary sub-scores: (1) motor arm left, (2) motor arm right, (3) best gaze, and (4) best language. These were chosen because motor, gaze and language functions have well-established neuroanatomical regions. We tested a general linear model (GLM) with SPM12 using each NIHSS sub-score as a covariate of interest, with age and gender as confounding variables. T-test was used to test for significance with two criteria (1) the p-value <0.05 (FWE corrected) and (2) the extended threshold ≥ 100 voxels.

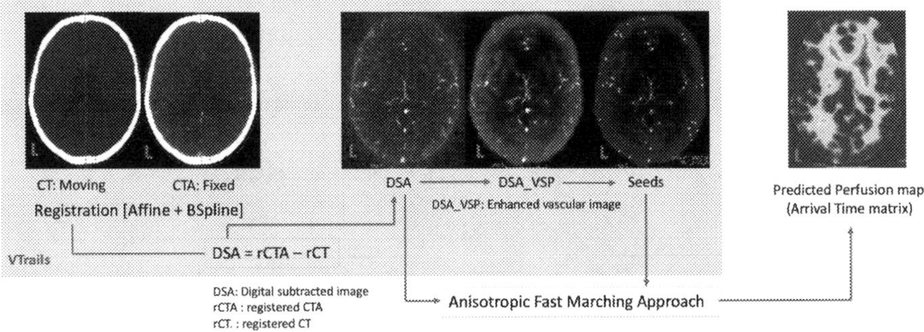

Fig. 1. Preprocessing steps in VTrails and the estimation of the predicted perfusion map.

3 Results

3.1 Longitidinal Analysis

From the 18 patients, we found an average correlation of 0.7893 (SD = 0.049, min = 0.6990, max = 0.8844). A significant correlation was found in every subject, see Table 1. Figure 2A shows two typical examples. In subject A07, the T-max map and the PPM highlight the ischemic core and penumbra covering almost all of the left hemisphere. In subject A16, the ischemic core located in the right frontal lobe can be seen in both maps. Note that we also estimated the correlation coefficients between the non-smoothed images. Similarly to the smoothed version, both modalities are highly correlated with an average correlation coefficient of 0.707 (SD = 0.031, min = 0.659, max = 0.7868). Using Spearman's rank test, we found no significant correlation between the spatial similarity index of PPM-and-Tmax with age (rho = −0.0548, p-value = 0.8290, see Fig. 2B, which is desirable as our PPM should be independent of age.

3.2 Cross-Sectional Analysis

From the four GLMs derived from 2110 subjects, our PPM mapped brain lesions to stroke symptoms in the expected regions. The left-hand motor score correlated with the right motor cortex and corticospinal tract (Fig. 3A; darker regions indicate a more significant effect). As expected, the laterality was reversed for the right-hand motor score (Fig. 3B). The best gaze score correlated more to the voxels in the right hemisphere (Fig. 3C). The best language score correlated with left perisylvian regions (see Fig. 3D). This suggests patients with left hemisphere stroke have a higher chance of having right-hand motor problems as well as problems with languages, moreover, patients with right hemispheric stroke will have a higher chance of having left-hand motor problems and visual problems, both of which match expectations.

Table 1. List of Spearmen's correlation between PPM and Tmax map in the 18 subjects, * = significant correlation, $p < 0.05$

Subject	Spearmen's correlation	Subject	Spearmen's correlation
A1	0.7856*	A10	0.6990*
A2	0.7529*	A11	0.7665*
A3	0.7817*	A12	0.8492*
A4	0.8237*	A13	0.7598*
A5	0.8146*	A14	0.8844*
A6	0.8131*	A15	0.7642*
A7	0.8444*	A16	0.8301*
A8	0.8238*	A17	0.7054*
A9	0.7648*	A18	0.7442*

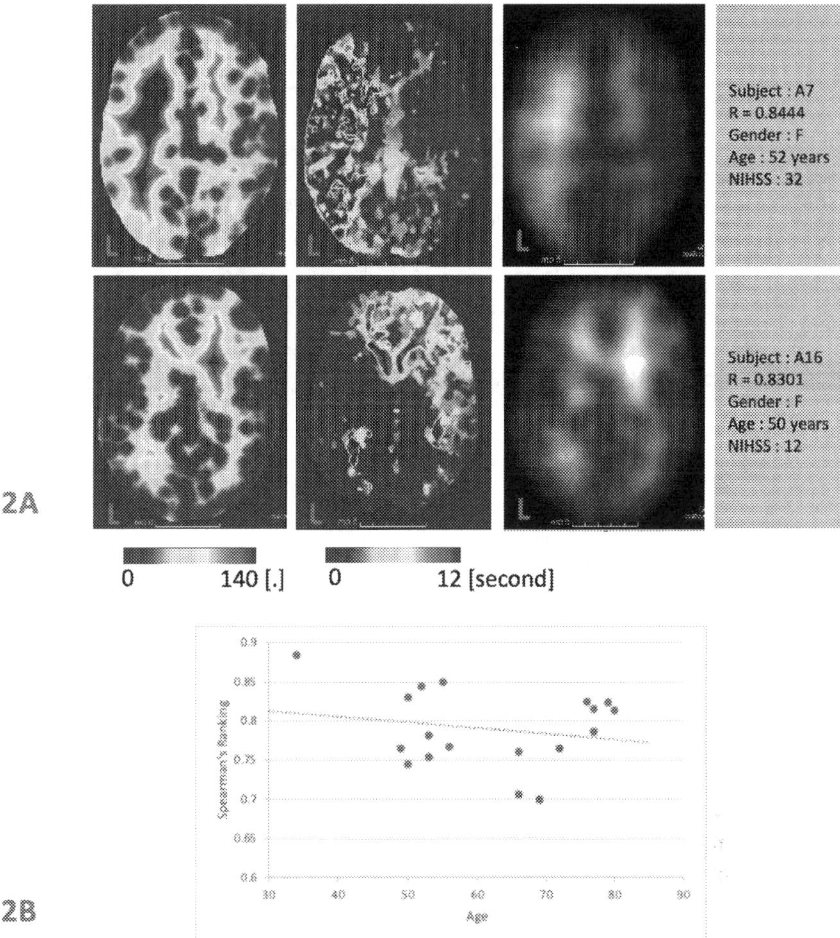

Fig. 2. 2A: Two typical examples of the PPM and the T-max map. Each row consists of three sub-figures, from left to right, the PPM, the T-max map, and the smoothed T-max map overlay on our PPM's smoothed version. In the predicted perfusion and T-max maps, dark red represents the area with a high risk of permanent brain damage, whereas blue represents the area with a low risk. The overlap map was created for illustrative purposes to highlight the overlap between two brain images. The units in the predicted perfusion and the T-max maps are dimensionless and seconds, respectively. Note that: L = left hemisphere. 2B: Spearman ranks plotted against age for all subjects. Each dot represents each subject's spatial similarity index (Spearman's correlation coefficient). The dotted line shows no significant correlation between age and the spatial similarity index between the two modalities (Color figure online).

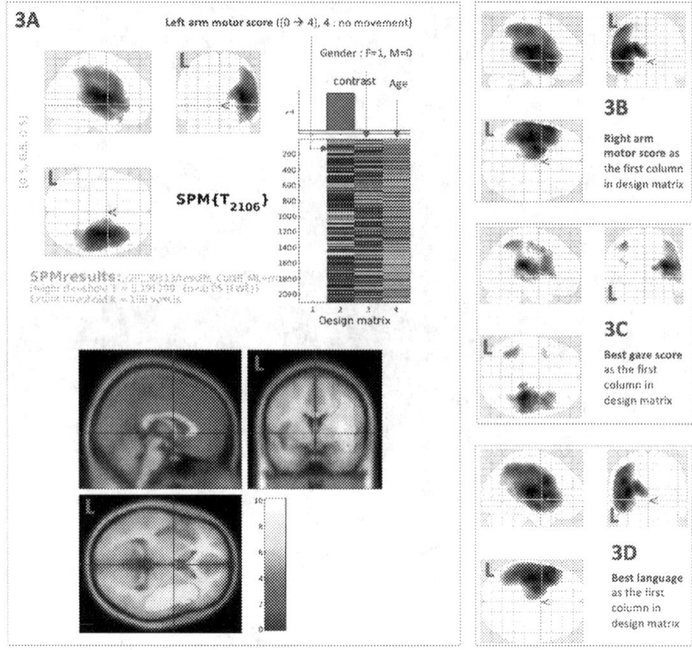

Fig. 3. Four GLM models in which different NIHSS subscores were used as covariates. 3A: Left-hand motor score, 3B: Right-hand motor score, 3C: Best gaze score, 3D: Best language score. Each section shows the brain in sagittal, coronal and axial views with a mean intensity projection of the voxelwise significance scores for each GLM contrast (darker = more significant). Section 3A also shows the SPM design matrix with the tested contrast over the variable of interest. L = left hemisphere.

4 Discussion

In this work, we presented a framework to generate a perfusion map constrained by physical and geometrical properties as an alternative to the traditional 4D perfusion map. Our PPM is generated from CT and CTA images, which can be acquired at the onset of stroke admission and are commonly available. In the eighteen patients with available 4D-CTP, we confirmed that our PPM was predictive of T-max maps from subsequently acquired 4D-CTP independent of subject age. We chose to compare our PPM with T-max since it is used to define the final infarct size and functional outcomes after recovery [21]. Moreover, in the cohort of 2,110 patients, the PPM correlated with stroke symptom scores in predictable, specific regions. Besides the lateralisation found in the contralateral motor cortex to the affected hand, we showed symptoms lesions maps associated with language and gaze (visual) problems, which is in line with the findings reported by Bonkhoff et al. [23], which used data collected within one week after stroke onset.

Like all lesion-symptom mapping analyses, we note that our results are constrained by the underlying vascular anatomy and potential clinical utility in situations where 4D-CTP is impractical. In our patient population, the cohort with plain CT and CTA was over one hundred times larger than the cohort with 4D-CTP. The aim of the work isn't to replace 4D-CTP; it is to provide a means of obtaining as high-fidelity an alternative from admission that relies only on admission scans (CT/CTA) as opposed to depending on additional scanning sessions. We mathematically derive PPM directly from CT and CTA images, which are the standard scans applied to every patient admitted to a stroke unit. Our PPM, an algorithmically derived estimation of the Tmax map, can provide clinicians with a continuous scale of brain areas with a high risk of cell death with no additional cost of having another brain scan or additional exposure to unnecessary radiation.

4.1 Conclusion and Future Work

To our knowledge, this is the first time the perfusion map was investigated on this large scale. Our PPM agrees with the T-max map generated from RAPID-AI software and highlights the brain infarction, which emphasizes the predictability power of our PPM. Although the number of patients with RAPID-AI images is still relatively low compared to the number we used in our GLM analysis, a statistically significant correlation between PPM and T-max was found in all subjects. In the future, we will address this limitation by performing the analysis in a large cohort or by using DWI as a surrogate for 4D-CTP, as it is more commonly acquired in hospitals.

Acknowledgements. CT, PB, SM, PW, PN, SO, and MJC are supported by the Wellcome Trust (WT213038/Z/18/Z). MJC, JT, and SO are also supported by the Wellcome/EPSRC Centre for Medical Engineering (WT203148/Z/16/Z), and the InnovateUK-funded London AI Centre for Value-based Healthcare. YM is supported by an MRC Clinical Academic Research Partnership grant (MR/T005351/1). JT is also supported by NHSX Ai Award and the Maudsley BRC. PN is also supported by the UCLH NIHR Biomedical Research Centre.

References

1. WHO website. https://www.emro.who.int/health-topics/stroke-cerebrovascular-accident/index.html. Accessed 5 June 2023
2. Saver, J., et al.: The "Golden Hour" and acute brain ischemia. Stroke **41**, 1431–1439 (2010)
3. Advani, R., Naess, H., Kurz, M.W.: The golden hour of acute ischemic stroke. Scand. J. Trauma Resusc Emerg. Med. **25**, 54 (2017)
4. Demeestere, J., Wouters, A., Christensen, S., Lemmens, R., Lansberg, M.G.: Review of perfusion imaging in acute ischemic stroke from time to tissue. Stroke **51**, 1017–1024 (2020)

5. Moustafa, R.R., Baron, J.C.: Pathophysiology of ischaemic stroke: insights from imaging, and implications for therapy and drug discovery. Br. J. Pharmacol. **153**, S44–S54 (2008)
6. Bandera, E., Botteri, M., Minelli, C., Sutton, A., Abrams, K.R., Latronico, N.: Cerebral blood flow threshold of ischemic penumbra and infarct core in acute ischemic stroke. Stroke **37**, 1334–1339 (2006)
7. SPM12 website. https://www.fil.ion.ucl.ac.uk/spm/software/spm12. Accessed 5 Mar 2023
8. Moriconi, S., Zuluaga, M.A., Jäger, H.R., Nachev, P., Ourselin, S., Cardoso, M.J.: VTrails: inferring vessels with geodesic connectivity trees. In: Niethammer, M., et al. (eds.) IPMI 2017. LNCS, vol. 10265, pp. 672–684. Springer, Cham (2017). https://doi.org/10.1007/978-3-319-59050-9_53
9. Stefano, M., Zuluaga, M., Jäger, H.M., Nachev, P., Ourselin, S., Cardoso, J.M.: Inference of cerebrovascular topology with geodesic minimum spanning trees. IEEE Trans. Med. Imaging **38**, 225–239 (2018)
10. Slicer website. https://www.slicer.org/. Accessed 5 June 2023
11. Perona, P., Malik, J.: Scale-space and edge detection using anisotropic diffusion. IEEE Trans. Pattern Anal. Mach. Intell. **12**(7), 629–639 (1990)
12. VTrails website. https://vtrails.github.io/VTrailsToolkit/. Accessed 5 June 2023
13. ITK website. https://itk.org/. Accessed 5 June 2023
14. Lee, T.C., Kashyap, R.L., Chu, C.N.: Building skeleton models via 3-d medial surface axis thinning algorithms. CVGIP: Graph. Models Image Process. **56**(6), 462–478 (1994)
15. Konukoglu, E., Sermesant, M., Clatz, O., Peyrat, J.-M., Delingette, H., Ayache, N.: A recursive anisotropic fast marching approach to reaction diffusion equation: application to tumor growth modeling. In: Karssemeijer, N., Lelieveldt, B. (eds.) IPMI 2007. LNCS, vol. 4584, pp. 687–699. Springer, Heidelberg (2007). https://doi.org/10.1007/978-3-540-73273-0_57
16. Benmansour, F., Cohen, L.D.: Tubular structure segmentation based on minimal path method and anisotropic enhancement. Int. J. Comput. Vis. **92**, 192–210 (2011)
17. El-Amin, M.F.: Fractional-Order Modeling of Dynamic Systems with Applications in Optimization, Signal Processing and Control, vol. 2, chap. 3, 1st edn. Academic Press (Elsevier), Cambridge (2022)
18. Zaro-Weber, O., Moeller-Hartmann, W., Heiss, W.-D., Sobesky, J.: Maps of time to maximum and time to peak for mismatch definition in clinical stroke studies validated with positron emission tomography. Stroke **41**, 2817–2821 (2010)
19. Wouters, A., et al.: A comparison of relative time to peak and Tmax for mismatch-based patient selection. Front. Neurol. **8** (2017). https://doi.org/10.3389/fneur.2017.00539
20. Campbell, B., et al.: Cerebral blood flow is the optimal CT perfusion parameter for assessing infarct core. Stroke **40**, 469–475 (2011)
21. Fainardi, E., et al.: Tmax volumes predict final infarct size and functional outcome in ischemic stroke patients. Ann. Neurol. **91**(6), 878–888 (2022)
22. Stroke National Institute of Health website. https://www.stroke.nih.gov. Accessed 5 Mar 2023
23. Bonkhoff, A., et al.: Generative lesion pattern decomposition of cognitive impairment after stroke. Brain Commun. **3**(2), 1–18 (2021)

Author Index

U. Baid et al. (Eds.): BrainLes 2023/SWITCH 2023, LNCS 14668, pp. 163–164, 2024.
https://doi.org/10.1007/978-3-031-76160-7

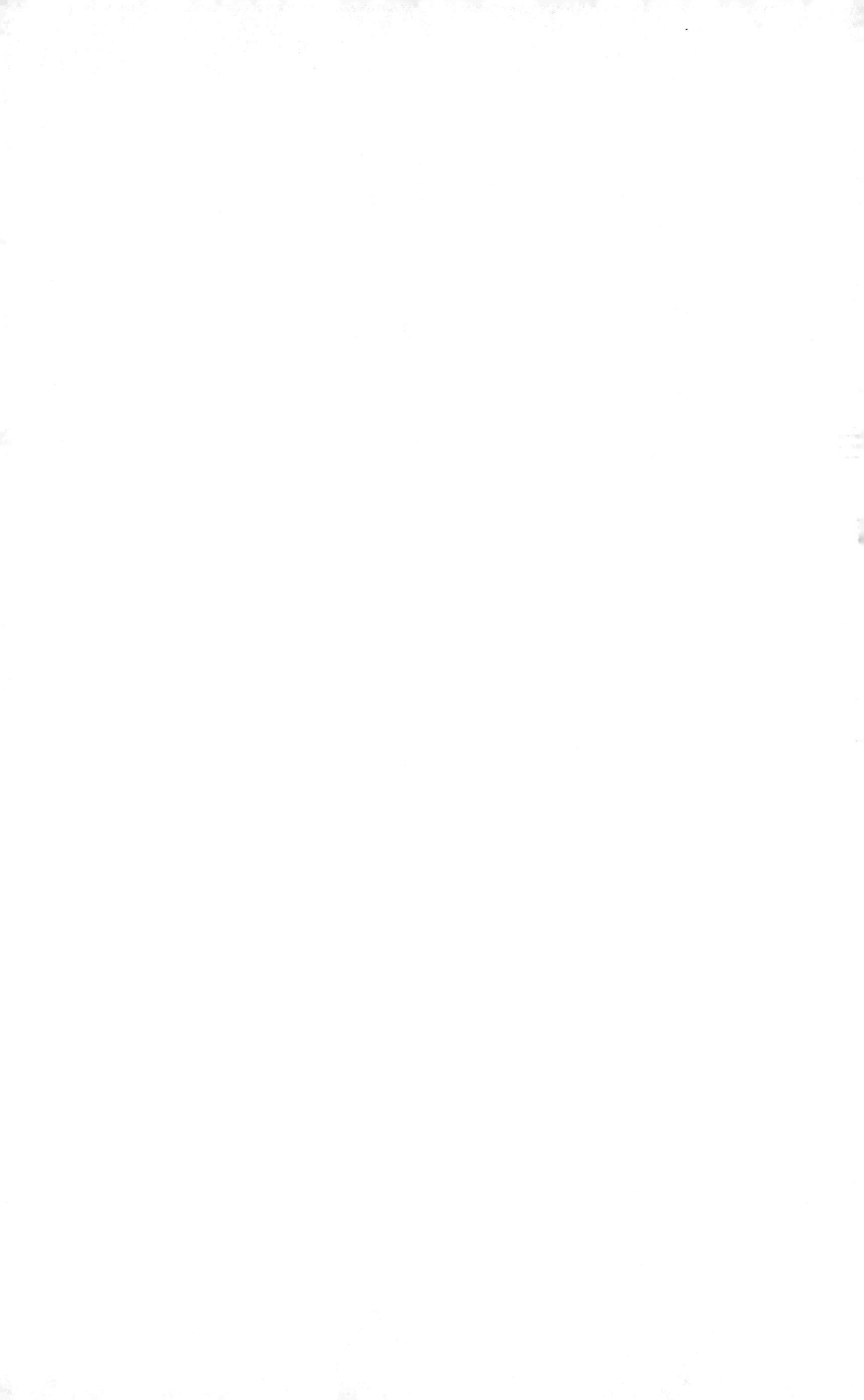